Prevention & Care

OF ATHLETIC INJURIES

Prevention & Care
OF ATHLETIC INJURIES

DR. DOUGLAS N. GRAHAM

"Look to your health; and if you have it, praise God,
and value it next to a good conscience;
for health is the second blessing that we mortals are capable of;
a blessing that money cannot buy."

~ Izaak Walton, 1653

Prevention & Care of Athletic Injuries

Published by:
FoodnSport Press

Visit us on the Web at http://foodnsport.com, or call us toll-free at (877) 811-4569.

Printed in the United States of America

Copyeditting: Kimberly Moranda and Susan Gast

Layout and cover design: Vickie Swisher

FoodnSport logo design: Janie Gardener

Project management, research, and additional writing: Andrew Perlot

Print ISBN: 978-1-893831-12-4
Ebook ISBN: 978-1-893831-03-2

DEDICATION

This book is dedicated to everyone who chooses to be physically active. May the joy you experience through fitness fun never be dampened by injury, or unnecessarily prolonged recoveries.

ALSO BY DOUGLAS N. GRAHAM

The 80/10/10 Diet, Grain Damage, Nutrition and Athletic Performance, Perpetual Health Calendar, The High Energy Diet Recipe Guide

TABLE OF CONTENTS

INTRODUCTION

A NEW LOOK AT PREVENTION AND CARE

With so many books on the market covering the prevention and care of athletic injuries, there is no need to write yet another unless an entirely new approach to this area can be introduced. This book provides such a unique perspective, while also offering the best of current advances in health and sports sciences. I hope you find that it becomes an essential resource and welcome addition to your sports and health library.

CORRECT THE CAUSE

At the heart of this book is a focus on strengthening the vitality of the human frame so that injuries are few and far between. Unlike traditional recommendations that tend to be based on the prevention and treatment of symptoms, it is my belief that viewing the body through a health-supportive, holistic lens will ultimately participate in creating a level of health that prevents injury and disease. Raising the consciousness of coaches and players to the degree that most injuries actually no longer occur is one of the goals of this book.

AVOIDING FAILURE AT THE WEAKEST LINK

If you were building a wagon wheel with sixteen spokes, you would want each spoke to be exactly the same length as the others, or else the resulting wheel would be out of round. Whether a spoke was too long, creating a high spot in the wheel, or too short, resulting in a flat spot, it would adversely affect the balance and overall functioning of the wheel. The same concept can be applied to prevention and care of injuries; no aspect is more important than any other, and the total program is only as strong as its weakest link.

We tend to enjoy activities that we consider ourselves good at, and to avoid those that we do not excel in. By practicing the activities that we are good at, we grow progressively better at them. We often ignore, and consequently get worse at, those activities that we do not excel in (when was the last time you did pull-ups?). Ignoring our weakest links makes the wheel go even further out of round.

Even though we often feel that focusing exclusively on our strengths will make our total program better, this is simply not true. Once again, picture the wagon wheel. If you had one spoke just slightly longer than the others, the wheel would be out of round and would not roll smoothly. If you were to further lengthen that spoke, it would only serve to distort the wheel further. In the same way, by overdeveloping your skills in one specific area, you diminish your capacity to be a well-rounded athlete. Furthermore, by ignoring (and consequently getting worse at) those activities that we do not excel in, we develop a greater likelihood of injury. Ignoring our weakest links ultimately weakens our capacity to excel fully in our chosen sport.

Prevention and care of injuries is an effort comprised of many facets, all of which are interdependent. Like any team, this concerted effort can be no more effective or efficient than its weakest member or link. No group can travel faster than its slowest member. The strongest members (links) are simply waiting for the weaker members to improve. When the weakest link is strengthened, the entire program functions better. By applying the weakest link concept, you can make the most progress with the least amount of effort.

"By overdeveloping your skills in one specific area, you diminish your capacity to be a well-rounded athlete."

CRUTCHES CRIPPLE

The old adage, "crutches cripple," applies fittingly to the world of sports injury management. If a perfectly healthy man were put on crutches for a month, forcing him to use only one leg, his unused leg would go lame. Similarly, using any lifestyle crutch unnecessarily—

"When we *correct the cause* by enhancing the lifestyle factors that create health—rather than attempting to prevent or treat symptoms—we will have made a quantum leap in our approach to health and sickness care."

whether for physical, nutritional, chemical, psychological, or other reasons—has a crippling effect rather than a health-enhancing one.

Rather than drink coffee to overcome tiredness, it's healthier for the body to get sufficient sleep. Instead of taking supplements to supply "missing" nutrients in the diet, it's healthier to eat whole foods that provide the full spectrum of nutrition.

Even recommendations of extended bed rest as a method of recovery from injury or surgery are rapidly coming to an end. Doctors and physical therapists have learned that recovery from almost all injuries is enhanced when patients resume physical activities as soon as possible. Sufficient rest is necessary, of course (see Chapter 7), but too much rest actually delays recovery, essentially functioning as a crutch, with less-than-optimal results. (To determine when you are ready to reengage in training following an injury, see the guidelines in Chapter 15.)

This book focuses on injuries, but the "correct the cause" directive applies to every aspect of lifestyle. When we *correct the cause* by enhancing the lifestyle factors that allow the body to create health—rather than attempting to prevent or treat symptoms—we will have made a quantum leap in our approach to health and sickness care.

YOUR AMAZING SELF-HEALING BODY

Cut your hand and it will likely heal all by itself. Break a bone and it too will heal by itself, without guidance or intervention from anyone. Of course there are times when intervention is beneficial, such as in life-and-death emergencies, but fortunately, these do not occur as often as we may think. Most of the time, the best method for healing wounds and injuries is simply to provide just enough rest, along with the other conditions required for overall health.

The body runs itself. It's a self-contained, self-healing, self-monitoring, self-repairing, self-organizing, self-creating, self-cleansing, and self-determining organism. Your body is designed to experience health, and in an effort to gain and maintain health, it is constantly adapting to the conditions, influences, forces, and substances to which it is subjected.

Vitality plays an integral role in health and healing. Individuals with low vitality heal more slowly than vibrant people. Often, low vitality is also associated with poor awareness. Staying healthy, alert, and aware are valuable assets when it comes to injury prevention.

Vitality can be expressed as "nerve force" or "nerve energy." Taking good care of your central nervous system is in fact taking care of your vitality and your overall well-being. Maintaining this nerve force requires sufficient rest, sleep, fresh air, sunshine, pure water, physical activity, and at least two dozen other facets of health. Below is a list of 32 elements of healthful living. See if you can add any elements to this list for yourself. All aspects of healthful living combine to create the ever-improving level of health that we are all striving for.

"Taking good care of your central nervous system is taking care of your vitality and your overall well-being."

FUNDAMENTAL ELEMENTS OF HEALTH

ARE YOU THRIVING OR SURVIVING?

Rate yourself, from zero to ten, in how well you meet your needs in each of the following areas.

_____ 1. Clean, fresh air
_____ 2. Pure water
_____ 3. Foods for which we are biologically designed
_____ 4. Sufficient sleep

_____ 5. Rest and relaxation
_____ 6. Vigorous activity
_____ 7. Emotional poise and stability
_____ 8. Sunshine and natural light
_____ 9. Comfortable temperature
_____ 10. Peace, harmony, serenity, and tranquility
_____ 11. Human touch
_____ 12. Thought, cogitation, and meditation
_____ 13. Friendships and companionship
_____ 14. Gregariousness (social relationships, community)
_____ 15. Love and appreciation
_____ 16. Play and recreation
_____ 17. Pleasant environment
_____ 18. Amusement and entertainment
_____ 19. Sense of humor, mirth, and merriment
_____ 20. Security of life and its means
_____ 21. Inspiration, motivation, purpose, and commitment
_____ 22. Creative, useful work (pursuit of interests)
_____ 23. Self-control and self-mastery
_____ 24. Individual sovereignty
_____ 25. Expression of reproductive instincts
_____ 26. Satisfaction of the aesthetic senses
_____ 27. Self-confidence
_____ 28. Positive self-image and sense of self-worth
_____ 29. Internal and external cleanliness
_____ 30. Smiles
_____ 31. Music
_____ 32. Biophilia (love of nature)

HYGIENE, THE "DO NOTHING" CURE

Much of this book applies the healing concepts of hygiene with the science and art of injury prevention and care. According to the philosophy of hygiene, the best results are often achieved by providing healthful conditions and letting the body's healing nature run its course.

The History of Hygiene

In the mid-nineteenth century, numerous doctors from around the world started questioning the use of harsh drugs, invasive procedures, stimulants, irritants, and caustic, toxic, or otherwise noxious substances as methods of "curing" patients. In fact, what is now recognized as the "modern healthcare system" was coming into vogue. Time-honored methods of healing, such as pure rest and fasting, were being tossed aside. Pills, potions, elixirs, ointments, tinctures, and remedies of all types were taking over.

A few doctors became ready to stop the madness and advocated ending the drugging of patients. One even performed experiments in which he gave his unknowing patients dosages of water-only "elixirs," along with placebo "medicines" made of bread rolled into pills. This brave doctor's hunch was proven valid as he watched his patients get well on bread pills faster than his patients given patent medicine did. Before long a new school of thought regarding health and healing, called natural hygiene, began to develop.

Hygiene is the science of human health, and named after the ancient Greek goddess Hygeia whose job was to watch over our well-being. In ancient Greece, those who were ill would often go to a temple to heal. There, the priests acted as the only doctors, and patients would fast for several days while living outdoors in the open air. They would take in nothing but water and do nothing but rest. Eventually, the patients would be put on a diet of primarily fruits and vegetables.

Around the mid-nineteenth century, doctors and other health practitioners began mimicking the ancient Greeks' manner of caring for the sick. They began intervening less often, and less intensely. They educated their patients in the care of the human body, and helped them to identify how they had become sick. They began to focus more on supplying healthful conditions and less on medical intervention. Often, they were called "quacks."

While traditional doctors made fun of their "natural" style of healing, the practitioners of hygiene were nonetheless developing a reputation for getting sick people well. They were often successful in working with clients who had been told by traditional doctors that nothing more could be done for their conditions. When these "incurable" patients regained their health, traditional doctors dubbed the turnarounds misdiagnoses or spontaneous remission, or they simply turned a deaf ear. Since hygiene offered no medicine or treatment other than supplying healthful conditions, it became known as the "Do Nothing" cure.

As stories of its success spread, Hygienic care became more accepted as a method of healing. Many famous practitioners of this method left their mark on society through the products or techniques they promoted. Breakfast-cereal mogul John Harvey Kellogg used these principles, as did famous nurse Florence Nightingale. Health pioneers such as Horace Fletcher, Sylvester Graham, Sebastian Kneipp, Arnold Ehret, and the customs of many other early Hygienists still influence healthcare practices today.

Kellogg popularized the concept of internal and external cleanliness in speeding the healing process. During the Crimean War, Nightingale became a celebrity when the press publicized her efforts to care for wounded soldiers and sanitize the military hospitals where they were recovering.

Fletcher promoted the "fletcherizing" of food: a process of chewing food thoroughly so that it is emulsified for optimum digestion. Graham (originator of the graham cracker) touted whole grains as health food and renounced the use of chemical additives. Kneipp was famous for a "Water Cure" that used hydrotherapy in conjunction with the principles of the "Do Nothing" cure. Ehret wrote extensively about creating health, with the bulk of his work focused on eating non-irritating foods that digested rapidly and did not result in the formation of mucus.

In more recent times, Dr. Herbert M. Shelton took the works of many of his predecessors and created the coherent body of knowledge known today as the Hygienic System. Dr. Shelton did so much work to promote hygienic care that many people still presume him to have been the originator of hygiene, and his name is still associated with the very word. From the 1920s through the 1960s, Dr. William Howard Hay released a series of popular books extolling the virtues of certain hygienic principles, specifically those of correct food combining. In 1985, Harvey and Marilyn Diamond exposed the world to more concepts of hygiene with their groundbreaking best seller, *Fit for Life.*

All of these health enthusiasts, plus many others who espoused a similar philosophy (for example, the proponents of exercise who became part of the Physical Culture movement) had one thing in common: their work was designed to help sick people get well. My desire is that the prevention and care methods described in this book do the same by helping people recover fully and vitally from exercise and training injuries.

DOING NOTHING, INTELLIGENTLY

Rest is not "doing nothing," as we may have been taught to believe; rather, it can and should be perceived as a valuable and pleasant activity. While we may act apologetically about resting when caught ("I'm sorry, I was taking a nap"), we should instead understand and appreciate rest as a necessary pleasure. The basic needs of human health are all pleasant experiences: rest, sleep, fresh air, sunlight, human touch, clean water, foods for which we are designed, and of course, physical activity.

To this day, some envious uninformed mainstream doctors continue to belittle the hygienic approach by calling it the "Do Nothing" cure. Hygienic doctors, understanding that intervention is not always beneficial and often works against the patient's best interests, respond by saying that they do nothing when nothing is called for. In fact, "doing nothing, intelligently" has proven in many instances to be one of the smartest moves that one can make when attempting to build one's health.

"The basic needs of human health are all pleasant experiences: rest, sleep, fresh air, sunlight, human touch, clean water, foods for which we are designed, and of course, physical activity."

DEVELOPING CONFIDENCE IN YOUR BODY

When we're feeling good and experiencing health, It's easy to expound on the hygienic value and logic of "attaining health through healthful living". This philosophy becomes much more difficult to abide when our personal health is challenged or loved ones fall sick. When people experience pain and distressing symptoms, the urge to intervene is profound. Only through seeing the effectiveness of hygienic principles in action can one gain faith in this time-proven healing system. Your body is designed to experience health, and to heal rapidly after injury.

The best results are commonly achieved when we simply provide healthful conditions, sit back, and let nature take its course. After experiencing successful results firsthand repeatedly, you will begin to develop confidence in your body's ability to heal itself, given the proper conditions.

REDUCING RISK: "THE THREE TS"

Most fitness activities are safer than ever due to the evolution of technology, training, and teaching.

1. TECHNOLOGY

Technological advances in equipment construction and materials have combined to make many physical activities safer today. Lighter yet more efficient padding, ergonomically designed equipment, and other technological advances have affected most sports activities, making them safer and often more enjoyable as well.

Equipment design modifications typically follow the injury trail. For instance, batting helmets in baseball were used sporadically more than seventy years ago, when players were getting hurt from hits on the head. Yet it wasn't until several decades—and many ear and head injuries later—that use of batting helmets with standard protective earflaps became commonplace. Nevertheless, even after-the-fact, such improvements are critical to the safety of athletes.

Improvements in design are often overlooked or quickly accepted and then forgotten by participants, coaches, and spectators, but they make a huge difference in reducing injury risk. Streamlined and better-designed equipment reduces the likelihood of many different injuries. All-weather running tracks provide safer footing than their cinder forebears. Modern tennis rackets absorb shock far better than did their predecessors. Bicycles have more efficient brakes for improved safety. Footwear has become specialized to meet the unique movement patterns of different activities. Foam pits and overhead rigs protect gymnasts from potentially-devastating falls.

Comfort, with a minimum loss of performance, is also a modern consideration, making physical pursuits both more accessible to the average person as well as more enjoyable and less likely to result in injury. Cushioned bicycle seats, soft easy-grip handles on weights, educational gear just for children, and entry-level fitness tools for beginning adults are prime examples of comfort combined with safety.

2. TRAINING

Athletes understand that injuries are their nemesis and create the worst of setbacks. The losses incurred as a result of injury are both financial and emotional. They can affect an entire career, while upsetting team performance.

"I can't take gym this week, coach, I hurt my shoulder," or, "I can't work out, I twisted my ankle" are common laments that need never be heard again. With today's improved understanding of well-rounded training principles, interruptions in training are unnecessary if injury does occur. The weight lifter with a bad back, the sprinter with an injured Achilles tendon, the bowler with a vision problem, the dancer who feels dizzy–all are being held back by their one weakest link.

Injury provides the opportunity to focus on aspects of training that usually receive insufficient attention. There is always *something* that you can do, regardless of the impediment that is seemingly holding you back. Since your weakest link restrains you the most, you will actually benefit the most by putting your efforts on strengthening it. Yesterday's sprained ankle meant two weeks or more off from training. Today's ankle sprain opens the door for flexibility, strength, and neurological training. Training today also builds up muscles and

"The more, the better" was the old motto for many athletes. This has wisely been replaced by "train smarter, train harder."

range of motion using specialized warm-ups and cool-downs, and step-by-step progressions that help athletes excel in their sport of choice without getting injured or reinjured.

Reducing the Chance for Reinjury

Repetitive injuries are no fun for anyone. We now know who is prone to such injuries, and why. Modern training and rehabilitation techniques have come a long way to help prevent repetitive injuries from occurring.

Multidimensional Cross-Training

"The more, the better" was the old motto for many athletes. This has wisely been replaced by "train smarter, train harder" by fit folks in the know. The difference comes down to cross-training. Cross-training not only reduces the boredom experienced by many die-hard sports enthusiasts who use only one activity for fitness, it also improves their performance in their chosen activity while reducing the likelihood of overuse injuries.

Time and again it has been shown that skiers who ski 48 weeks per year and cross-train during the other 4 weeks outperform those who ski 52 weeks per year. For those of us who do not play sports for our living, cross-training provides exceptional value when used as a regular part of the workout routine.

Five Aspects of Fitness

No sport is one-dimensional, as virtually all activities require at least some ability in all aspects of fitness—muscular strength, muscular endurance, cardiorespiratory, neurological skill, and flexibility. Some activities demand a relatively equal balance of all five fitness aspects. The argument about whether the person who is exceptional at one aspect of fitness is a greater athlete than the person who excels equally at all five (and vice versa) is timeless.

3. THE THEORY OF INJURY-FREE MOVEMENT

Theory today offers an improved understanding of athletes' learning and health capabilities, which helps make education and instruction on how best to avoid and care for injuries more effective and efficient.

You will see the following important themes highlighted again and again throughout this book:

- Correcting the cause by strengthening weak areas and avoiding crutches
- The body as self-healing and self-correcting, and
- The importance of providing proper nutrition, rest, recovery, and other elements for thriving.

Part 1 — Injury Prevention

If you want to be fit for a lifetime, then fitness must be a lifetime activity.

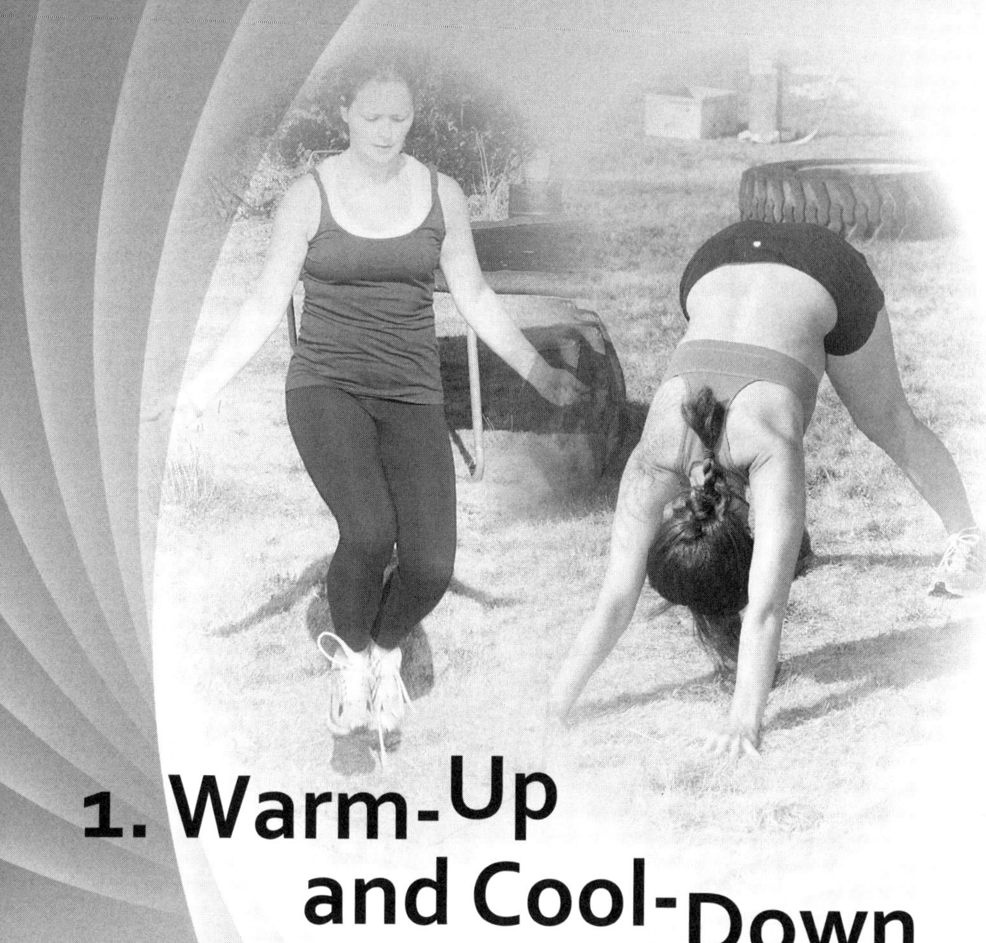

1. Warm-Up and Cool-Down

Perhaps the most important factor for preventing athletic injury is consistently incorporating a warm-up and cool-down in every workout routine. Warming up correctly allows you to make the most of your fitness sessions by preparing the muscles, connective tissues, and other relevant structures for the more vigorous and challenging activity to come, which reduces the chances of injury. Cooling down properly is equally important as it reduces the likelihood of stiffness, soreness, and other post-workout problems. Both warming up and cooling down promote injury prevention, quicken short-term recovery, and set the stage for the body to heal any injuries that might occur.

"Warming up and cooling down promote injury prevention, short-term recovery, and aided healing from injury."

THE VALUE OF ROUTINES

Developing a sense of routine in warm-up and cool-down procedures is important. There are infinite possible approaches to these parts of your training sessions, yet certain key bases must be covered, no matter how it is done. A routine is useful for many reasons, including but not limited to developing and establishing: comfort, reliability, confidence, and the ability to evaluate your progress successfully, as well as orderliness, and comprehensiveness.

OLD FRIENDS MAKE FOR COMFORT

If you want to be fit for a lifetime then fitness must be a lifetime activity. Warming up and cooling down should become like old trusted friends for you. The more comfortable you are, the less you'll be in a rush to leave them; as you gain confidence in their value for you, you will want to spend more time in their company.

RELIABILITY

Like a true friend, you will come to rely upon thorough warm-up and cool-down routines to help you in your training. Their value becomes more noticeable over time. Eventually, anyone wishing for a lifetime of fitness will have such assurance that their warm-up and cool-down are valuable, that they would never even think of forgoing them.

CONFIDENCE

When caring for people with many different types of injuries, I was often told, "I thought I was ready, but I wasn't." Effectively performed warm-up and cool-down routines will breed self-assurance in your skills much as a cyclist's regular practice of shifting gears creates confidence in his ability to select the right one for the terrain. You will know with certainty when you are ready to switch from one gear to another, because you will have developed the ability to evaluate your progress.

EVALUATION

Warming up and cooling down provide an excellent opportunity for evaluating how you feel and how your body is responding to the demands you have been placing on it. During warm-up, you can safely reassess the day's workout plan to be sure it's in alignment with what your body and mind are telling you.

During cool-down, you can develop a realistic assessment of your recent performance and begin to plan your recovery and even your next fitness session. If you feel great at the end of a workout, you might realize that you could have given more effort. If you feel exhausted, you might realize that you simply pushed yourself too hard. (These topics are covered in greater detail in Chapters 5 and 6.)

> **"If you feel great at the end of a workout, you might realize that you could have given more effort. If you feel exhausted, you might realize that you simply pushed yourself too hard."**

ORDERLINESS

There is a natural order to the warm-up and cool-down. Usually when we are about to initiate physical activities, we are coming from a relatively sedentary state. Bringing yourself to a point where you are ready for lively exertion, while minimizing the risk of injury, requires a sequenced approach.

Admittedly, being organized can probably be carried too far. But there is a lot to be said for good organization and the thoroughness that usually accompanies it. There are key points to every warm-up and cool-down, and milestones that should be noted as they are passed. By monitoring your progress in a sequence of increments, you will have taken the necessary precautions to prepare for your upcoming activity. It's a good feeling to know you've "covered your bases" and that all precautions have been taken in preparing for your upcoming activity, even if it is the high-stress mechanics of full-out exertion.

When warm-up and cool-down are pursued in this fashion, the transition from sedentary to active and back again is steady and gradual. By using increments you can effectively "test the water" of your readiness in warm-ups as well as carefully guide yourself back from intense exertion in cool-downs.

COMPREHENSIVENESS

Most people know offhand what foods they eat and household goods they use in a typical week, yet many still use a checklist when going to the grocery store to avoid coming home from shopping only to realize that an important ingredient or other necessity was forgotten. With your warm-up and cool-down, leaving out a step can often result in injury or unnecessary delays in training or recovery, either of which can be far more inconvenient than merely having to go back to the store.

Some injuries can be life-changing, and rarely is it for the better. Be sure to use a warm-up and cool-down checklist until you have it memorized and are positive that you are being thorough.

MAKING A CHECKLIST

When warming up or cooling down, once the body gives the "all systems are go" response to one increment, it is appropriate to move on to the next. If you get a warning signal that you are not yet ready to move on, increase the time and energy spent on that segment until you are.

Below are checklists of key points you will want to focus on in your warm-up and cool-down sessions. These will be explored in detail throughout the rest of the chapter. You can tailor the checklists for your workout regimen as specifically and in as much detail as you like.

Warm-Up Checklist

1. Start gently. Starting off too quickly, or too aggressively, will likely result in injury.
2. Take your time. A thorough warm-up should take 20–30 minutes, but can take longer.
3. Begin with general warm-up activities before focusing on warm-up movements specific to your chosen activity of the day.
4. Remember that the goal of warm-up is to raise core temperature; feeling warm, sweating, increased rate and depth of breathing and

so on are attempts at staying cool—they do not indicate that true body warm-up has occurred.

5. Gradually increase the intensity of your movements throughout the warm-up in order to eventually arrive at the expected tempo of your training session.
6. Pay attention to what you are doing.
7. If not fully hydrated, drink water during the warm-up to facilitate hydration.
8. Mobilization of the joints, range-of-motion activities, and general and specific movements are all part of a comprehensive warm-up. Stretching is most effective during the cool-down.
9. Once the warm-up is completed, it is best to transition directly into your fitness activities. If you must pause in between, remain somewhat active and use additional clothing so as to prevent unwanted cool-down, muscle stiffness, or other undesirable effects.

Cool-Down checklist

1. When activity finishes, discourage rapid cool-down by utilizing extra clothing to hold the heat.
2. If weather makes cooling down difficult, insert brief periods of inactivity, such as stretching, intermittently throughout the cool-down.
3. Do not foreshorten the cool-down. Allow for about one minute of cooling (minimum) for every ten minutes of exercise. Cool-down can easily last for thirty minutes after a long training session.
4. Be certain to address your hydration requirements as soon as possible during the cool-down.
5. Take your time. A rushed cool-down is never satisfactory, and will diminish its effectiveness and increase your recovery time.
6. Pay attention to what you are doing. Cool-down is a common time to make silly errors that can result in unnecessary injuries.
7. Cool-down is the most effective and safest time for stretching.
8. Bring your workout to a close gradually by reducing the intensity of activity from all-out to complete rest over the duration of the cool-down.

9. Utilize walking and other non-jarring, rhythmic activities in the cool-down in order to help prevent blood pooling.

WARMING UP AS WE GET OLDER

As we age, the need for warming up and cooling down generally increases, especially if we continually attempt to reach the levels of intensity that we achieved when younger. The muscles, joints, connective tissues, and other parts of the body need more time to achieve full readiness for activity, and take longer to cool down after exertion.

A five-year-old child will probably need a much shorter warm-up before playing tag than a fifty-year-old will. As you age, you will want to consider three main possibilities for modifying your approach to warming up and cooling down:

1. Go about the entire process in a less-hurried fashion. Take more time with each aspect of the warm-up and cool-down to really appreciate the nuances of each.
2. Flesh it out: add variations to "accessorize" your existing warm-up and cool-down. This method is the natural outgrowth of mastery of any skill. As we become more familiar with the basics of any process, we become more adept at adding flourishes, variations, and nuances.
3. Incorporate completely new elements or convert segments from your exercise sessions into the warm-up and cool-down instead. The options are limitless. You will often find that extending the warm-up and cool-down in this way is surprisingly enjoyable.

FOCUS ON THE NOW

The easiest way to get hurt while exercising is to be thinking about something other than what you are doing. In fact, this is one of the quickest paths to the emergency room. During warm-up and cool-down, practice keeping your mind focused on the present, putting any worries or preoccupations of the day away, as they really are of no concern while you are exercising. It's extremely important—and gratifying—to stay in the moment while exercising.

THE WARM-UP

The main purpose of a warm-up is to prepare the body for vigorous activity. By exposing your body to gentle exertion that progressively increases, you condition and prepare yourself for actions that will be even more intense. By the end of the warm-up, all aspects and facets of your physical capabilities should be ready for action.

Another major purpose of warming up is to prepare the body for high-level activities. When a person is active near the limits of his or her physical abilities, the mechanical stresses on the body soar. During such "high-stress mechanics," the weakest link—be it muscle, bone, ligament, tendon, fascia, or other tissue—becomes exceptionally prone to injury. One of the primary aims of the warm-up is to prepare the body for such high-stress mechanics.

"Warming up" is commonly accepted to mean raising the core body temperature by 1°F. Though extremely objective, this definition often proves impractical because most people have no convenient way to measure body temperature during exercise. Fortunately, there are other ways to ensure that you are ready for lively exertion while minimizing your risk of injury. A sequenced approach to warming up is the safest and best way to transition your body from sedentary to active.

WHAT A WARM-UP IS NOT

Time is short for most people, and motivation to spend it warming up is often not very high. Therefore, it's important that your warm-up not be diluted or wasted by unfocused effort.

A Warm-Up Is Not Stretching

Warm-up activities are designed to overcome the body's ability to maintain its core temperature. Stretching cannot do this. Stretching is an important part of a proper cool-down, but holds no place in warm-up activities for most sports. Practicing any of the following will make for an effective warm-up: joint mobilization, neurological skills, mild range- of-motion movements, or joint- and muscle-function facilitation drills.

A Few Possibilities For Your Warm-up

Jogging, bear crawls, juggling, balancing on an unstable object, skipping, lunges, jumping rope, arm and ankle circles, dribbling a basketball, back bridges, bodyweight squats, olympic lifts with an unweighted barbell or PVC pipe, plank holds.

A Warm-Up Is Not 1–2 Minutes

The function of the warm-up is to overcome the body's ability to maintain resting homeostasis[1] and to enter into a state of exertive homeostasis. It's actually physiologically impossible to raise one's core temperature in just a few minutes; the body is too well-equipped to throw off extra heat. According to most exercise physiologists, it takes a minimum of twenty to thirty minutes or more of warm-up activities to raise core temperature by one degree. This means that proper warm-up sessions should take close to thirty minutes on average before you consider them concluded.

"Proper warm-up sessions should take close to 30 minutes on average before you consider them concluded."

A Warm-up Is Not Sweating, Being out of Breath, or Feeling Warm

The start of perspiration does not so much represent a rise in body temperature as much as an attempt by the body to *prevent* such a rise. Even though a proper warm-up makes you feel warm long before it is over, sweating, feeling warm, and being out of breath are not indicators that it's time to move on to the workout. These are simply signs that the body is attempting to cool and refuel itself.

1 Homeostasis is essentially the body's attempt to maintain its chemistry and physiology within an acceptable range of parameters. Temperature, blood pressure, pulse, respiration, blood chemistry, hormone production, and so forth all function optimally when kept within guidelines predetermined by the body.

HAVE FUN AS YOU WARM UP

Warm-up drills and skills need not be boring or unpleasant, and we can turn our warm-ups into play. I usually have the most fun during warm-ups, and sometimes extend my warm-up activities so that they make up the bulk of my entire fitness session.

BUILDING A COMPREHENSIVE WARM-UP

There are many ways to create an effective and comprehensive warm-up. The sequence and activities you select will provide many possible variations. Still, you'll want to include the following key elements whether your warm-up is general or customized for a specific sport and skill set.

Getting in the Mood

Mentally transitioning from being at home or at work to being in an exercise environment can take time. During the warm-up, you have the perfect opportunity to switch your mindset to the activities ahead. While doing the gentle exercises of the warm-up, you can plan and focus on the activities and precautions you wish to cover in your fitness session.

"While doing the gentle exercises of the warm-up, you can plan and focus on the activities and precautions you wish to cover in your fitness session."

Taking as Much Time as You Need

When preparing to workout with others, I've noticed that many people finish their warm-ups almost before I've started my own. Maybe you've had a similar experience when playing tennis or basketball with friends. You needn't lose face by saying that you need more time. You can ask to extend the start-up practice, or suggest that you all do a little more warming up.

Ultimately, only you will know how much time you need, and how badly you need it. You will be the one to suffer with injuries if you go all-out in an unprepared state. Until your warm-up is complete, it is not truly safe to engage in full-intensity activities.

If you're looking for inspiration to be methodical with your warm-ups, consider how the Olympians and the pros approach warming up. We can see how deeply these athletes concentrate and prepare for their given sport in every performance.

They arrive early and warm up before spectators even begin to fill the stadium. Then, behind closed doors, they make sure to keep warm and stay focused on their pending performance, doing one more short warm-up just before the event. Unless you arrive very early to a game, you won't see the warm-up. Take a cue from the Olympians and pros and take the time you really need to warm-up;you'll likely not only develop your training ability but also your self-regard as an athlete.

Range-of-Motion Activity

Range of motion should be explored fully during the warm-up, but not through an emphasis on stretching (which should be saved for the cool-down). Activities to encourage full range of motion should use extremely gentle and small movements, gradually building into larger ones as the body warms and the muscles become more supple. For example, arm circles can start with a small circumference that increases in size.

Slow-Speed Walk-Throughs

Learning a skill in slow motion is a desired option in many sports. The slow-speed walk-through is a valuable learning tool. One of the best ways to stave off injury from high-stress mechanics is to perform them in slow motion as part of the warm-up. In addition, you will be practicing and perfecting skills crucial to your sport. Once high-stress mechanics skills are learned, performing them in slow motion as part of the warm-up is an excellent method of practicing and perfecting the skill's nuances.

Difference Between Warm-Up and Actual Play

Giving a percentage value to the level or degree of exertion is a method of differentiating between warming up and full-on, all-out play or exercise. For each person, the numbers may be a bit different, and they will vary as well depending upon the point in the work-out at which they are performed. At the start of a warm-up, movements might be done at one-quarter speed, eventually moving up to half-speed perhaps halfway through the warm-up. Three-quarter speed would be done at the three-quarter point of the warm-up. One would not actually work out at full speed until the warm-up was almost completely finished.

General Aerobic Activity

The majority of sports and exercise routines can make use of similar basic aerobic warm-up activities such as jogging, jumping jacks, skipping, or jumping rope.

TIME FRAME OF A COMPREHENSIVE WARM-UP

Safe, effective, and comprehensive warm-ups consist of two distinct phases. Phase 1 prepares the body for general exertion (as described in detail above), while Phase 2 (described in detail following the time frame) emphasizes preparing the body for the specific activity to follow.

Phase 1 (Basics): 5–10 Minutes

This phase begins when you engage in a general range of motion and aerobic elements. Every physical activity poses slightly different requirements upon the body. Some, such as running, call for a relatively specific and limited range of movement, whereas others, such as racquetball, will require far more.

When the muscles are going to be used in a repetitive and predictable fashion, using the first ten minutes of your warm-up to perform actions that mimic those of your sport—with less intensity—will be sufficient. For example, running relatively slowly would be a very good warm-up for a thirty-minute jog.

Phase 2a (Sport-Specific): 10–20 Minutes

For athletic pursuits that require greater range of motion, this second phase of the warm-up should be more intense and sport-specific.

For example, if the activity is going to include running but will also demand changes in direction, jumping, or other movements (such as football), it would be wise to use this segment to gradually build speed or experiment with relatively short bursts of speed, but without going to maximum running exertion levels.

Phase 2b (Skill-Specific): 20–30 Minutes

If you are intending to go all-out in your workout, at least another ten minutes of warm-up is required. This period should be designated for using the specific skills and drills of the sport to be played. Sport-specific warm-ups can be done as isolated movements or as groups of skills linked together in a series.

SPORT-SPECIFIC WARM-UPS

Once the general activities have been performed, it is time to get more specific by introducing the distinctive and unique movements that are integral to your sport or activity. The benefits of performing sport-specific activities during a warm-up include readying the muscles and brain for the more intense iterations to come, a reinforcement of game-critical skills and neural pathways, and a reduction in your risk of being injured during actual play.

Example of a Sport-Specific Warm-Up: Running

Many people think that moving the legs in a basic "mock running" motion sufficiently warms up the body for a run, but it really doesn't. Perhaps this perception persists because running is a relatively straightforward exercise, especially when compared with the complex ranges of movement required for many sports. Nevertheless, there are several factors to consider when prepping for a run.

The muscles and type of muscle fibers you will use depends greatly upon whether your run is uphill or downhill, fast or slow, and on even or uneven terrain of grass, rock, or asphalt. Arm and shoulder girdle action also play a strong role in running, hence the muscles, joints, and connective tissues of this area should also be fully warmed up prior to running with intensity. Even if the running surface is perfectly flat, core stability is still used in running to some degree, therefore, the muscles and abilities involved in generating core stability should also be prepared during the warm-up for almost every type of activity.

SKILL-SPECIFIC WARM-UP

If you were a basketball player, the general warm-up for all days would likely be the same. Much of the sport-specific warm-up would also be similar, though there might be some variations based on the planned activities for the day. The skill-specific warm-up would likely vary greatly from day to day, as each day's fitness demands would be very different.

"The skill-specific warm-up provides an excellent opportunity for psychological preparation, which can be practiced at almost full intensity, without the stresses of game time."

Some days you might focus on offensive plays, some days on defensive plays. Some days the emphasis would be on shooting, other days it might be on ball handling, and on others, it might be primarily on basketball-related fitness training.

There is more than physical readiness developed in the skill-specific warm-up. Mental alertness must also be enhanced. The skill-specific warm-up provides an excellent opportunity for psychological preparation, which can be practiced at almost full intensity, without the stresses of game time. Skill-specific warm-ups can be used as a dress rehearsal and to pay great attention to detail. Skill-specific warm-ups can focus on run-throughs many times until near perfection is achieved.

Example of a Skill-Specific Warm-Up: Basketball

Staying with the basketball example, we can infer that different types of warm-ups would be used on different days. The days that focus on offensive plays would likely include large amounts of footwork and agility skills with related warm-up drills performed. The defensive-focus days would include strength training geared especially toward control of momentum, and would include tactical skills.

On the days that emphasize shooting, particular care would be taken in warming up the fingers, hands, wrists, forearms, elbows, arms, and shoulders, with somewhat less emphasis put on lower body warm-up. On days that ball-handling skills were worked on, the warm-up would be sure to include the various muscles and ranges of motion required for passing and receiving, along with copious quantities of neurological skills. And fitness days would require their own specialized approach to warming up.

WHEN TO END THE WARM-UP

Your core temperature is up, your focus is sharp, you are feeling flexible, and you have covered the basics and specifics for your chosen activity—in short: it is time to begin your training in earnest. But what if you're not quite sure your warm-up is completed? If completing your warm-up routine according to your watch does not give you the confidence that you are ready, there is still hope. In this case, testing the waters to see if you're ready to move on to the workout is an excellent choice.

If running is your intended activity for the day, you could run relatively rapidly for just a few steps, perhaps from one geographic marker to the next. Alternate your pace from fast to slow between them.

You could also try going "fast, faster, and even faster" for short distances, alternating with slow jogging. If after several attempts you feel absolutely ready to commit to your workout in full, go for it. If you are not convinced that you are ready, or if for some reason you still don't feel ready, add in more warm-up procedures, perhaps at a relatively high degree of intensity.

Once you think you have finished your warm-up, try performing your skill at a high level. For instance, if you are heading out for a run, you will likely have started by walking, eventually building into a jog during your warm-up. As you're building up speed in your jog, make some other movements: go sideways and backwards, take some cross-steps, add in a few jumps—eventually you should be able to tell if you have finished warming up by your sense of "all systems go"—and you'll know you are ready to move into full-blown running.

The sense of readiness reached after fifteen to thirty minutes of warm-up is completely different than the feeling of anticipation you get when you first begin. You will feel—and be—much more in the rhythm of your chosen activity. Your concentration levels will rise and using maximal exertion will seem effortless and natural. At this point, the warm-up can be concluded.

Unfortunately, for most people, this feeling is not achieved until about fifteen or twenty minutes into their actual workout, well after they have completed their foreshortened warm-up. This overlap between "finishing" the warm-up and starting the workout is a time when all too many injuries happen. Extending the warm-up is always preferred over injury or even compromised performance.

THE COOL-DOWN

Perhaps one of the most underrated and underemphasized aspects of fitness sessions is the cool-down. The body must make many physiological adjustments in order to change temperature. It is advantageous to slowly bring the fevered state achieved in fitness pursuits back to normal ranges. Sometimes referred to as the warm-down, this relatively short part of each fitness session is essential for ensuring speedy recovery and for minimizing the risk of post-workout stiffness, soreness, and other problems.

As with warming up, cooling down is most effective when performed in stages. Toward the end of your training session, gradually taper into the cool-down by reducing the intensity of your exercise. Downshift your pace as you would gears: from fifth to fourth, fourth to third, and so on. An effective cool-down can reduce the likelihood of future injuries by enhancing the recovery time of the muscles through increased delivery of vital minerals such as potassium, thus improving the quality and structural integrity of tissue developed.

BLOOD POOLING

During exercise, the volume of blood flowing to the muscles in use greatly increases. Blood vessels dilate to allow for the greater volume.

Take time during the cool-down to allow the blood vessels to constrict, bringing blood volume back to normal. The pooling of blood in muscles after a workout discourages muscles from fully flushing their toxins, reduces the efficiency with which muscles can uptake glucose, and increases the potential for blood clots.

Aided Release of Muscle Toxins

Lymphatic vessels run parallel to almost all of the blood vessels. Exercise increases the rate of flow within the lymphatic system, the primary "pump" of which comes from external changes in pressure. Toxic wastes from muscle cells are released into extracellular fluids and picked up by the lymphatic system to eventually be released into the blood. Pooling of blood in the muscles results in an overall reduction in blood flow to any given area and is paralleled by an equal reduction in lymphatic flow. This reduction of blood and lymphatic drainage results in slower pickup of cellular metabolic waste products, one of the primary factors that can slow recovery times from exercise.

Reduced Potential for Clots

Pooled blood sits relatively still in engorged vessels, creating an increased propensity for clotting. A blood clot within the blood vessel is known as a thrombus. A thrombus can result in a stroke. A well-rounded and extended cool-down greatly reduces the risk of a thrombus or stroke occurring.

An Influx of Glucose Delivery

In order for muscles to recover after exertion, they must be exposed to sufficient blood glucose. Blood pooling reduces overall glucose delivery, as the blood lacks mobility. A thorough cool-down improves both drainage of muscle toxins (i.e. waste products of cellular metabolism) and delivery of nutrients to the muscle cells, greatly enhancing muscle recovery and reducing risks of subsequent injury.

STRETCHING

The cool-down is the best time to incorporate stretching into your exercise program. When fully warmed up, all tissues are more elastic and willing to stretch, making tearing or other injury less likely. Joint fluids have also warmed and are runny, allowing the joints to better yield their fullest range of motion.

Stretching should not be rushed and is most useful when performed in stages. Suddenly stopping your workout and moving into a lengthy stretching session without incorporating periods of movement can be almost as jarring as failing to warm up properly. Cooling down too quickly increases the likelihood of blood pooling, muscle soreness, and muscles stiffness.

By working in movement, you also extend the cool down period, and therefore the amount of stretching you can do while still being relatively warm, which increases the efficiency of your program.

In hot weather this is less of a concern, but it becomes easier and easier to cool down too quickly as the weather gets progressively colder.

After an hour of running, you'll benefit more from alternating between brief periods of stretching and walking than you would from stopping on a dime and beginning a 15-minute stretching session. As your pace slows, your heart rate will come down and your walking can be slowed even further. Continue this pattern until you have stretched all of the muscles involved in your activity and cooled down properly.

Working General and Specific Flexibility

During your cool down stretching, it's a good idea to keep in mind the need to increase both general and activity-specific flexibility.

Piano players exemplify specificity when it comes to flexibility. They practice their reach constantly, and eventually are able to easily reach spans that had previously been impossible for them. Piano players generally sit when playing, so their general flexibility is not challenged, but their hands can become far more flexible than average.

Every activity poses unique flexibility challenges. Overall or general flexibility should be a lifetime fitness goal. There is definitely some truth to the old saying that you are as young as you are flexible. Before putting too much attention on specific flexibility persuits, make sure you're maintaining good overall flexibility.

Jarring Increases the Need for Stretching

The need for stretching is also partially determined by the type of stresses you're putting your body through.

You may have noticed that there are many books filled with stretches for runners but few on stretches for swimmers. Have you ever wondered why? While swimmers also need to stretch to reach their fullest potential, they generally can get away with doing less stretching than runners because they are less prone to jarring in their sport. Certain receptors in the muscles and tendons respond to jarring with an overall shortening of these fibers.

This makes the muscles and tendons tighter and more prone to pulling and tearing. Therefore, the more jarring you are exposed to in your chosen activity, the more stretching should play a role in your cool-down.

THE ROLE OF WEATHER IN YOUR COOL DOWN

Atmospheric temperature, wind, and other environmental factors can cause you to cool down too quickly. On the other end of the spectrum, extremely hot and muggy weather can make for a very slow cool-down. In both instances, there are techniques to modulate the pace of the cool-down.

Use Clothing, Shade, Showers, Etc.

Clothing helps to keep you warm by holding in body heat. In cool weather, you can slow a cool-down with the judicious use of clothing. It's often wise to wear a bit more clothing than you think you need after exercising to ensure that you cool down comfortably and fully.

In very hot weather, it is not uncommon to be perspiring freely twenty or even thirty minutes after your fitness session has been completed. In such situations, look for shade or cover; your cooling off will be far more rapid than in full sun. Finding a breeze will also help.

If the humidity is not high, try wetting your head or skin and let the evaporation cool you slowly but surely. In calm, sunny conditions with high temperature and high humidity, it might be necessary to take a cool shower or a dip in cool water to finally complete the cool-down.

WHEN TO START THE COOL-DOWN

While many injuries occur due to poor judgment (and judgment can be strongly affected by tiredness, among other factors), many injuries are also due to a lack of connective tissue integrity. A well-timed cool-down can prevent injuries that occur from overextending a workout session beyond safe limits.

Tired? Mind Wandering? Time to Call It a Day

Pay attention for when a fitness session reaches a point of diminishing returns. Although there is value in sheer endurance, especially if that is the primary goal of your fitness session, as peak performance tails off so do the benefits to be gained from that session. When tiredness increases, there is a directly proportional increase in the propensity for injury due to compromised technique.

"It is important to notice when a fitness session has reached a point of diminishing returns."

A sure sign of fatigue is when it becomes difficult to maintain your focus on the matters at hand. When your mind wanders and you start thinking about what you need to be doing after you finish exercising, it is time to call it quits and start the cool-down.

HOW LONG SHOULD A COOL-DOWN TAKE?

Extending the cool-down long enough to allow blood flow to return to pre-exercise distribution levels is extremely important. Aim to cool down for approximately one minute for every five to ten minutes that you were exercising. Temperature, humidity, intensity, duration, and frequency of exercise are just a few of the factors that affect the length of the cool-down required.

As a rule, it is better to err on the side of caution, extending your cool down rather than cutting it short. Longer cool-downs that include plenty of stretching have been shown to greatly reduce the amount of post-exercise stiffness, delayed onset muscle soreness (DOMS), and general aches and pains that accompany training. It's well worth your while to extend your workout session by an extra few minutes with a cool-down.

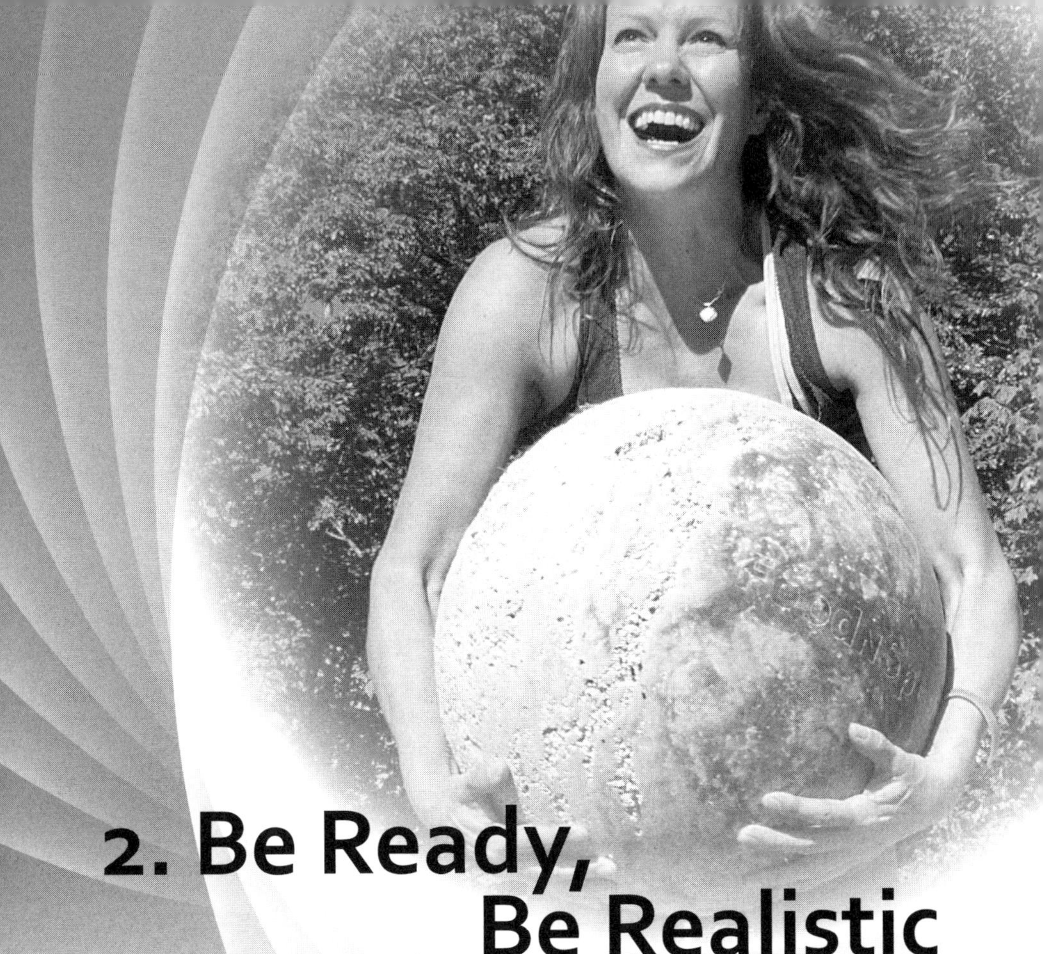

2. Be Ready, Be Realistic

In my hometown, I was considered a pretty good skateboarder as a kid. I used my skateboard to go everywhere. The terrain was pretty flat where I lived, though, so when I went skateboarding for the first time near my cousin's house in the Catskill Mountains, I was simply not ready to handle the steepness of the slope. On the first hill we attempted, I found myself accelerating and totally out of control.

I was heading straight downhill, unable to turn, and gaining speed. Eventually I was pitched off the skateboard and onto the asphalt. Other than bruises and abrasions, I wasn't badly damaged, but it could have been much worse, as the road we were skating on intersected a major highway at the bottom of the hill. When caring for clients with injuries, their stories often have a similar theme. They tell me: "I thought I was ready, but I wasn't."

SAFE BEATS SORRY

How many times have you wished you could turn back the clock in order to avoid an injury that has already occurred? Try as we might, it simply cannot be done. We have to learn to live with our mistakes as well as with our injuries.

At worst, injuries can be fatal or impose permanent setbacks on our training and our ability to enjoy fitness activities. At their best, injuries still present a temporary inconvenience, one that everyone would rather avoid. The pain, rehabilitation, and revision of one's training schedule make injuries unwelcome at any time.

"Try as we might, we simply cannot turn back the clock. We have to learn to live with our mistakes as well as with our injuries."

If you are not sure about the safety of a given situation, choose a more secure option rather than be sorry. Opportunities to incur injury are hidden in every activity. When you sense danger you are always smart to avoid it. Learn to trust your inner voice of reason.

WEEKEND WARRIORS

Most of us enjoyed fitness activities as children, and many of us continued them throughout our school years. But when work, family life, social responsibilities, hobbies, home maintenance, and other time constraints begin to intervene, our fitness usually suffers. Eventually, we may only have time for fitness on the weekends. Weekend warriors often emerge in these circumstances, thinking they can be healthful by cramming a week's worth of fitness activity into just one or two days a week. The body reacts differently to sporadic and intense bursts of activity than it does to regular exercise, and the injury rate among weekend exercisers proves it.

When you are physically active every day, there is a certain calm assurance that you don't have to fit all of your training into one session. There is always tomorrow. You can plan your workouts so that you train in different aspects of fitness on different days, letting your body recover healthfully. But when you only have one or two days per week to stay fit, there is a strong temptation to up the intensity or duration to unrealistic levels.

There is an urgency to your activity, which may also cause you to condense the warm-up in a dangerous and vain effort to "maximize results" through your training session. Those who succumb to the urge to condense their workouts—making them more intense—usually pay with unnecessary injuries. The injuries only serve to set them back in their training.

If you must be a weekend warrior, be safe and be smart. Extend your warm-ups and your cool-downs. Choose activities that fit your abilities, and realize that without constant practice, ability levels will steadily decline. Try your best to find at least a few minutes each day to maintain your fitness and skills using specific warm-up activities so as to get the most benefit from your weekend workouts.

SKILL-LEVEL STAGNATION

"If you don't use it, you lose it" is one of the most time-honored and accurate expressions in sports. Skills that are finely honed throughout a sport season are easily lost through disuse and deconditioning, leaving us vulnerable to injury. Oftentimes, as we mature, many of the skills we developed as children become rusty as well, and we can no longer take them for granted.

Refamiliarize the Body

We cannot simply take up right where we left off when it comes to fitness activities. While we don't ever fully forget how to perform skills such as bicycle riding, bowling, or hitting a tennis ball, most of the fine-tuning is quickly lost.

To have exquisite reflexes in your chosen activity requires that you perform it with relative frequency—at least several times per week or more. Even if you are coming back to your sport after only a short time away, this still holds true. The finely tuned skills that we have developed by the end of a season are easily lost again through disuse.

"It is better to be redundant rather than negligent in your exercise preparation and warm-up."

A friend of mine was a ski instructor and a very good skier. On the first day of the season, before anyone else was allowed on the mountain, ski patrol and ski instructors were invited for a day of skiing. On her very first run of the season, going far too fast for full control, my friend made a slight miscalculation and caught an edge. Her run ended in a high-speed crash and injury that required fourteen hours of reconstructive knee surgery in order to give her a chance of recovering mobility. Her knee was never the same. She couldn't walk for almost a year. Skiing remained out of the question for over a decade and she could never ski aggressively again.

It's better to be redundant than negligent in your exercise preparation and warm-up. When reintroducing activities from your past, nothing is lost by taking an extra week or two to review. Being safe always beats getting hurt.

"I Used to Be Able To..."

None of us like to lose our abilities. When the world closes in on us in any way, we feel as though we are losing our personal power. As Joni Mitchell put it perfectly in her famous song, "You don't know what you've got till it's gone." When our physical abilities wane, whether from lack of use, injury, or the accumulated impact of lifestyle abuses, we feel the loss.

"When our physical abilities wane, whether from lack of use, injury, or the accumulated impact of lifestyle abuses, we feel the loss."

One day, my nieces and I were playing on the family trampoline. An uncle of mine, not much older than myself, was watching but declined to get on the trampoline when offered a turn. Instead he said some of the saddest words I have ever heard, "I used to be able to jump on the trampoline, but not anymore." I felt very sorry for him and vowed I would do all that I could to prevent myself from ever having to utter the words "I used to be able to."

Accurately assessing your abilities is important. Too many people overreach their grasp, thinking their skill-level is higher than it really is, only to be rudely awakened by injury. Though your pride may be somewhat dashed when you start out with the beginners in your attempt to regain former and partially forgotten skills, reacquainting yourself thoroughly with prior skills reaps many rewards. Your friends and family will give you far more credibility for being prudent and uninjured than for being reckless and spending time in the emergency room.

INACCURATE ASSESSMENT OF PRESENT SKILLS

In order to keep your skills developing, it is important that you push yourself, but it must be done in safe and reasonable increments. Many people feel that they must keep up with the competition, no matter how good the competition is. The truth is that there will always be people who are more talented than you are, at almost everything that you will ever do. If you find yourself in a group whose skill-level is above yours, attempting to stay with them is likely to lead to injury.

I remember very clearly a day I went snowboarding with a group of friends from Colorado, some of whom were professional snowboarders. I was so excited to be able to keep up with them, as I was a relative beginner at snowboarding. My skills had been developing rapidly, and I was feeling confident. On one run, everyone decided to go fast. My experience was thus far mostly limited to slow runs with lots of turns—it didn't include going fast and straight downhill. Nevertheless, I went for it, feeling exhilarated and proud that I was able to keep up. Everything was going fine until I saw a restraining rope across the snow, hung about chest-high.

It wasn't until I tried to swerve out of harm's way (something that everyone else in the group did almost effortlessly) that I realized how deeply I was in over my head. I had accumulated far too much speed to have any control. The rope almost bent me in two. Fortunately I wasn't hurt, but my pride certainly was. I had learned a valuable lesson. Knowing yourself and staying within your abilities are reliable rules for success when it comes to physical exertions. Only Superman can jump to the top of a tall building in a single bound. For the rest of us, it is smarter to avoid injury and take the stairs.

GROSS- AND FINE-MOVEMENT SKILLS

Getting on a bicycle after a long time off is not especially challenging, but riding it through a tight course that demands perfect control at slow speeds would be all but impossible. If you haven't played tennis in a few years, you will likely remember most of your favorite shots, but not be able to execute them with accuracy.

It's unlikely you will be able to get your serves in, or hit them with the speed that you used to muster. In these instances, the gross-movement patterns (those that require the largest muscle groups) are still working fairly well, but the fine-movement skills (those that require finesse and rely upon the coordinated efforts of many smaller muscles) simply will not function as effectively as when they were regularly practiced.

When assessing your abilities regarding any activity requiring finesse or coordination, be sure to consider both your fine- and gross-motor skills. If you do not set your sights too high, you will not set yourself up for disappointment. If you give yourself time to regain your fine-motor skills, you will likely find that you can play as well, or better, than you have been playing in your mind's eye. Forcing yourself to reach benchmarks you're not prepared will often lead to injury or otherwise strain your mind or body.

PROGRESSIONS

Watch children as they methodically learn a new skill at a skateboard park. First they perform the skill in miniature, and usually in slow motion, as many times as they need to until they feel comfortable. Then they do it bigger or faster. Eventually they build the skill up to full size and full speed. Learned properly, they make the skill look easy, the result of the hundreds or thousands of practice attempts that were performed away from the watchful eyes of spectators.

One of the best methods for making smooth and rapid headway during the skill-learning process is the liberal use of progressions. Progressions are the building of a complex skill by adding one movement at a time. When I was working as a trampoline coach, I stumbled onto a system of teaching that used progressions only. Once I showed my students the progressive relationship between one skill and another, they quickly caught on.

"One of the best methods for making smooth and rapid headway during the skill-learning process is the liberal use of progressions."

They loved my system because it seemed to them that they were teaching themselves, and in many ways they were. I loved using the progression system because it almost guaranteed that no one on my team would get hurt. (None of them ever did get hurt during all the years that I coached.)The system worked so well that in just four years, each member of the team went from being a rank beginner to a national champion.

Using progressions has many benefits, including building a skill base, reducing the likelihood of injury, increasing the understanding of movement patterns, and enhancing enjoyment and creative potential.

Building a Skill Base

When skills are learned in a step-by-step fashion it is relatively easy to progress without risk. It's important to understand all of the steps, and not to skip any of them. Physical prowess develops somewhat like building a pyramid. The larger the base of support, the taller the pyramid can be. If you build a solid base of skills, your fitness progress can be almost infinite.

Reducing the Likelihood of Injury

You're much more likely to experience an injury or accident if you attempt to perform skills without mastering the prerequisite progressions. As you master one step, the next becomes more apparent and more viable, always keeping your safety zone large.

Increasing the Understanding of Movement Patterns

As we master skills, it becomes easier for us to "accessorize" them. For instance, when learning to cartwheel, it is usually all you can do to survive it and land on your feet. With practice, though, you can learn to do the cartwheel with pointed toes, straight legs, even with a smile. With even more time and practice, you can learn to do cartwheels in either direction, one-handed, or ending on one leg only. Eventually, you could learn to do "dive" cartwheels and even to perform cartwheels on a balance beam.

However, if you started off by trying to learn the cartwheel on a balance beam, it would be a recipe for disaster. Learning a skill through progressions not only makes for a much safer experience, but also likely gives you a much fuller understanding of the movement patterns related to that particular skill.

The ability to embellish any skill is a good demonstration of your progress in learning that skill. Many people find that when they begin a new physical pursuit, the instructions and experience initially go by in a blur. Their awareness is being challenged almost to the limit. For example, when first learning to ride a bicycle or in-line skate, beginners must focus attention closely on what they are doing. In fact, if you were to ask beginners what they see while bicycling or skating, they would likely tell you that it is all they can do to focus directly ahead and not crash.

With practice, however, they will soon gain confidence and develop their abilities. And as their skills are honed, their peripheral vision will increase as well. Soon enough, the bicyclist will be able to look left and right while riding just as the skater will be able to look at a friend and wave.

There is a saying, "amateurs practice till they get it right, professionals practice till they don't get it wrong," and it accurately sums up the shade of difference that can make or break a performance. Regardless of the conditions or situation, professionals get it right a high degree of the time. Before you can consider a skill mastered, you should learn many variations of that skill.

Embellish it in different ways. Practice until you can do the skill well, even in unfavorable conditions. True mastery through the use of progressions will prove to be the safest, most enjoyable, and most varied method for learning.

Enhancing Enjoyment and Creative Potential

Though the beginning stages of any learning process can be somewhat tedious, we all relish the feeling of finally mastering a skill to the point where we can show it to someone else. Using progressions allows the learner to experience that happy feeling with increased frequency.

In my trampoline classes, I generally taught twisting skills in quarter-turn progressions. (Some students could learn faster, in half turns, but they lost nothing by mastering the quarter turns. Some students were slower learners, and had to learn in eighth-turn progressions.) With every quarter turn mastered, the students were elated. After years of using this technique, they were just as excited to add an extra quarter turn to a triple twisting move as they had been to add the same increment to their half twists.

An important point to keep in mind is that people learn at different speeds. You may require more steps than someone else to learn the same skill. Be patient with yourself. Ultimately, enjoyment, variety, and skill mastery will help you to prevent injury by increasing your awareness and by developing your body with sport-specific abilities.

LEAD-UP SKILLS

The proper use of lead-up skills in creating readiness for activities is almost an art form in itself. Related to progressions, lead-up skills are those abilities that you have already mastered and that will bring you to a state of readiness for performing more challenging skills. The more thorough and effective your preparations, the greater the likelihood you will remain injury-free throughout your fitness sessions. There are many ways that lead-up skills can be used to aid you in this endeavor.

Run Through Basics as a Warm-Up

The use of lead-up skills as a regular part of your warm-up is somewhat similar to a musician warming up through the practice of scales. Although these are basic skills, they are integrally related to the more complex movement patterns that you will perform when you go all-out. Review the basics, from easiest to ever more difficult, as a routine facet of warm-up. With each type of anticipated daily activity, there are different lead-up skills from which to choose.

Fine-Tune the Basics

One of the comments commonly heard about professionals in any field is that they make it look easy. What they do is not easy, it is just that they have spent an incredible amount of time practicing and perfecting their skills. In order for high-level skills to work, the fundamentals must be perfected. At the level of high-stress mechanics achieved in professional sports, if all movements aren't correct according to the laws of physics, an accident, injury, or poor performance is bound to happen.

Mastering the basics is an ongoing job. Many of the world's top professionals continue to practice basics until the end of their lives, constantly striving toward perfection. They see the benefits of practice, and know that the better they get at the basics, the better they will become in their most complicated performances. Our goal may not be to become a professional in our athletic pursuits, but we will reap the same benefits as the pros if we model ourselves after them in terms of practice.

"Mastering the basics is an ongoing job. Many of the world's top professionals continue to practice basics until the end of their lives, constantly striving toward perfection."

Practice does not make perfect. You only get better at what you practice. If you are practicing an error repeatedly, you get better at making that error. Only perfect practice produces perfect performance. Use lead-up skills to continue to practice perfectly every day.

Increase Focus

Some people count to ten in order to regain their calm when they have become upset. With practice, eventually they can achieve that calm state by counting only to nine. Over time, and with an aware mindset, counting to eight will suffice. With years of practice, counting to seven, six, five, four or three will do the job. Eventually just the inhale that initiates the count will be enough for the person to regain a state of total calm.

Running through lead-up skills works the same way in that it gives the performer a chance to focus on the finer aspects of the more difficult challenges to come. There are different types of lead-up skills. For example, you might find that practicing single pirouettes is extremely valuable before doing double pirouettes on the dance floor. Mechanical errors are more obvious as the level of mechanical stress rises. While you may be able to control a poor pirouette without losing balance, doing a double will likely show you that you are out of control, in no uncertain terms.

Some lead-up skills bear little resemblance to the advanced skills they can evolve into. We all pretended to be "wheelbarrows" as children, walking on our hands while our partners held our ankles near their waists and pushed us around. Gymnasts use this strength and skill to walk on their hands unassisted. Basketball players use the same movement to push the basketball when performing the chest pass. Swimmers, martial artists, and anyone who uses pushing as part of their fitness routine benefited by the simple lead-up of doing the wheelbarrow. There is even fitness apparatus on the market today so that you do not need the assistance of a partner to perform this valuable lead-up drill.

By using lead-up skills to prepare for working out, your muscles will be warmed, your joints will be lubricated, and you will be more limber overall, protecting you from injuries commonly associated with tight muscles, tendons, and stiff joints.

BUILDING READINESS

Learn to respect the importance of readiness when your goal is to be as fit and as injury-free as possible. Following is a tool for building readiness that will help you gauge the degree to which you are truly prepared.

Perfect Performance at Level Green

In the United States, the slopes at a ski resort are traditionally described as easy, moderate, or difficult via the designated markings of green circles (easy), blue squares (moderate), and black diamonds (difficult). Many skiers push themselves to see if they can "survive" the more difficult slopes, even though they will likely do so with poor form and occasional spills. It's not uncommon to see spectacular falls in which skiers' gear trails out on the snow behind them: poles, skis, and sometimes even goggles or a hat. Spectators riding the lifts refer to such a scene as a "yard sale." No one wants to be involved in a yard-sale spill; the embarrassment is nothing next to the bruises one takes home.

A pro skier I know taught me that he starts every ski session by taking a few runs on the green slopes, attempting to ski them perfectly. If he makes what he considers to be even the slightest mistake, he does the entire run again. Only after he makes three perfect runs in a row on the easiest slope does he move up to the blue runs and begin the process anew.

In any sport, it is a good idea to lock in a mental picture of yourself performing perfectly. By beginning each workout with the easiest skills and truly mastering them, you will help solidify this perfect mental picture. If you attempt to move on to more difficult levels too rapidly, not only will you cheat yourself of the pleasure of experiencing mastery, you also will inhibit your likelihood of progressing when performing at top speed, as well as increase your likelihood of getting injured.

Know Yourself and Know Your Limits for Exceptional Performance

To truly know your limits requires a lot of motivation and just as much practice. In the passion and enthusiasm of engaging play, it can be tempting to push yourself beyond your ability to perform safely. Rarely will you get away with exceeding your ability to withstand high-stress mechanics. We risk serious injury when we attempt to perform in ways that exceed our abilities or readiness. Following are two examples of understanding one's limits. As extraordinary as the accomplishments of these two men are, they still kept themselves within the zone of their known abilities.

Rudi Carti, a client of mine, is a personal trainer in Aruba. He and another personal trainer friend had a conversation about doing abdominal crunches, at which they both thought they were very talented. The friend asked Rudi if he thought he could do one thousand crunches in a row. Rudi didn't reply, but on his lunch break that day he found out that he could easily perform three thousand crunches in an hour. Later in the day, Rudi bet his friend he could do the thousand, and more. He did eighty thousand in a row. Later that year, Rudi performed 151,000 abdominal crunches in forty-eight hours, a world record.

A dear friend of mine, Dr. Timothy Trader, used to be a stunt man in the movies. One day he was asked to ride a motorcycle under an 18-wheeler, a very tricky and dangerous stunt indeed. When he instantly agreed, some people were surprised. They did not know that he had practiced this skill a great many times in the past and that he felt fully confident that he could do it successfully.

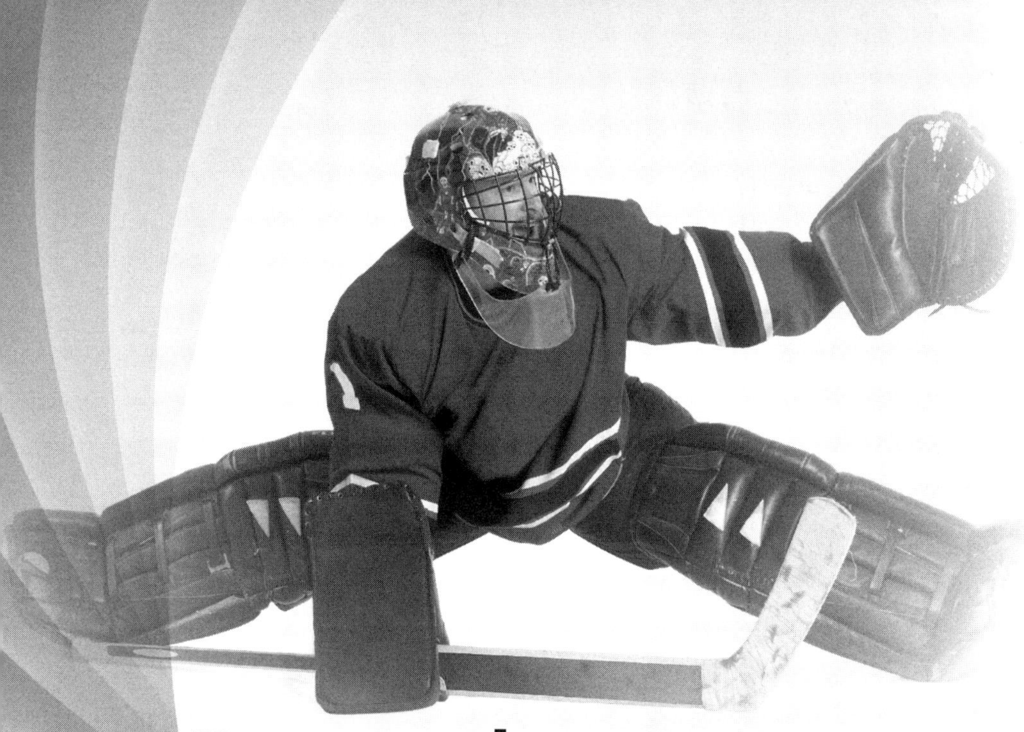

3. Protective Gear

I once watched a television program about sporting accidents that showed a race car accident in which the driver crashed head-on into a wall while going more than 200 miles per hour. The car went airborne, flipping and spinning wildly as it also burst into flame. When it landed, it rolled repeatedly—more times than I could count. The car totally disintegrated except for the safety frame. The driver? He walked away from the accident completely unscathed. That is protective gear in action.

Safety equipment is one of four major influences affecting your ability to train injury-free, along with coaching techniques, nutrition, and lifestyle. Using protective athletic gear generally makes sports far safer. But you have to use it to reap the benefits; by the time you realize that you need it, it is often too late. There is no valid reason to resist using appropriate safety gear.

Protective athletic gear is commercially available today for virtually every part of the body. Wearing it is simply an issue of self-respect. Get used to wearing gear in practice and when game time comes, it will feel normal and not encumber your performance.

Play Defensively

Always play with your best interests in mind. Play defensively, in a manner that makes it difficult for the other players to accidentally or even intentionally hurt you.

"Protective athletic gear is commercially available today for virtually every part of the body."

The Other Guy Can Be Unpredictable

As much as good sportsmanship is a part of every game, not everyone plays by the same rules. Sometimes people are mean. Sometimes they lose control of themselves. Protective gear can be a blessing when limbs and egos collide.

SPECIALIZED PROTECTION

HEAD

Head injuries are almost always serious, and are to be avoided at all costs. If a helmet is made for your chosen sport, you should likely be wearing it. You might even consider starting a trend by wearing a helmet for activities where its use is not yet the standard. Ten years ago, not one snow skier in a thousand wore a helmet. Today, almost 10 percent wear them and the number is rising.

Forty years ago, no one wore a helmet to play ice hockey. When the first guys started using them, it was considered unmanly. Today it is considered reckless to play ice hockey without a helmet, and the use of one has become mandatory in organized play, for all ages and abilities.

Always Wear a Helmet

One beautiful autumn afternoon years ago, I was riding my motorcycle home from college. I was going rather slowly down a quiet side street when I saw an oncoming car gradually veer into my lane. I considered my options. As the car drew nearer, I could see that the driver was totally focused on her passenger. I knew then that I was in trouble, and I jumped from the bike.

Being a gymnast with training in how to avoid injury in a fall, I rolled like a log down the road. As my head banged again and again on the asphalt I thought, "thank God I am wearing a helmet, thank God I am wearing a helmet."

They Don't Transplant Heads

"No one in history has ever survived decapitation."

~ Prof. Rozalind A. Gruben

Not Much Different Than a Watermelon

I have been told that watermelons will burst from about the same amount of concussive force that it takes to break open a human skull. While there are stronger parts of our skulls that protect us in a typical fall (the back is thickest), certain areas of the skull are very delicate indeed (such as the temple). If you wouldn't do it to a watermelon for fear of it bursting, don't do it to your head.

If in Doubt...

Always wear a helmet. Always wear a helmet.

EYES

There are few parts of the human body, if any, that we would be willing to live without. Certainly I cannot think of one. Topping the list of vital human body structures are the eyes. Though you can live without them, the body treats the eyes as one of the most important structures. Even in cases of severe starvation, the eyes are not damaged.

Your Eyes are Worth Protecting

I don't enjoy wearing protective goggles, nor do I imagine that there are many people who do. But I keep in mind that most protective athletic gear has been created only *after* a need for it has been repeatedly demonstrated. And I prefer to stay injury-free. For the sake of your eyesight, wear eyewear when it's called for. Damaging or losing your vision is devastating, but it's only inconvenient to wear goggles on occasion. You look far "cooler" with two eyes and goggles than you do with an injured eye.

Don't Wait Till You Need Them

As with helmets and head injuries, it is too late to put on protective eyewear by the time a bug, finger, branch, or piece of sports equipment lands in your eye. Being proactive is your best option.

TEETH

Teeth are easy to damage, but so easy to protect. Generic rubber mouth guards are inexpensive and often all that is needed to protect you from having a toothless grin.

An example of how unexpectedly teeth can be injured occurred when I was first learning to surf at about age nine. I was standing on the beach at the water's edge, waiting for my board to wash ashore with the incoming surf. I bent down to pick it up when it came close, not noticing the incoming wave had lifted the board and was propelling it toward me. The nose of the board hit me in the teeth before I knew what was happening. To this day, one of my front teeth is darker than the other, and I consider myself lucky to have escaped so lightly.

Mouth Gear Protects Your Teeth and Face

Mouthguards not only protect you from breaking teeth, they also protect you from the likelihood of doing serious harm to your lips and cheeks. The soft tissues around your mouth are easily damaged when compressed between hard or sharp objects such as teeth. For any activity where there is potential for contact with other people or equipment, a mouthguard is a sensible choice.

HANDS

My wood shop teacher in grammar school had only nine and a half fingers, having lost half of one in a wood-shop accident. Fortunately, few fitness activities present such overt dangers to our hands. Most of the hand injuries we experience during fitness pursuits come as bruises, abrasions, or blisters. Since we use our hands for almost everything we do, injuries to the hands are extremely inconvenient. It's not worth being uncomfortable with a blister or cut for a week or more when a small measure of protection can help you avoid it. Taping is one effective option for protecting your hands (and is discussed in detail later in the chapter). Gloves are another excellent choice; they are easy to put on and provide superb protection.

Sport-Specific Gloves

Protective gloves come in a variety of designs for different sports, including thick boxing gloves that protect the knuckles and finger bones, the dry gloves of a scuba diver that keep water out, and weightlifting gloves that prevent painful blisters. Today's gloves are comfortable, stylish, and extremely functional. In many activities, gloves give such an improved grip that they can enhance your performance. If gloves are made especially for your sport, you should likely be wearing them when you participate. The first time my bicycling gloves kept my hands from being torn up by asphalt, I was convinced to always wear them.

WRISTS

Wrist injuries can range from mild to extreme. The milder injuries are generally nothing more than wrists being sore from unaccustomed use and stress. For instance, should you start a program of daily push-ups, your wrists might "complain" slightly for the first few days. But by being gentle with your pace, your wrists will soon accommodate the new activity.

It is possible to sprain a wrist, but not common. Rather, severe injuries to wrists often involve a broken bone. Breaks at the neck of radius (the bone that leads down to the thumb) are quite common, as are breaks of the other bone of the forearm, the ulna. Both types of breaks are easily avoidable through the use of protective gear.

Wrist Guards

Modern wrist guards designed for in-line skaters do an excellent job of protecting wrists in many sports. If you are learning a new sport or skill where a hard fall is likely (as in skating, skateboarding, snowboarding, and the like), shield yourself from injury with wrist guards.

ELBOWS

Ever hit your "funny bone" and laughed it off? This mild damage to the ulnar nerve is usually not serious. However, falling on the tip of your elbow can easily result in a fracture, and is an entirely unnecessary accident.

Elbow Pads

Once again, the popularity of in-line skating can be credited for spurring technological advances in protective athletic gear. Soft, thick, and ineffective elbow pads of the past have been replaced by sturdy, thin, and streamlined protection designed for in-line gear. As with wrist guards, if you are a beginner, learning new skills, or entering into competitions where you will be pushing your ability limits, wear elbow pads. You can also choose to wear them as a matter of habit.

KNEES

I was walking in my hometown one day when I saw a teenager ride his bicycle into oncoming traffic. I have no idea what he was thinking, but the minivan driver that hit him was definitely not at fault. The boy was thrown about fifteen feet into the air and landed on the tarmac on his hands and knees. I won't sicken you with the details, but he was severely injured.

Another time, I was watching a skateboard competition in which a skateboarder took a similar fall. However, because he was wearing protective knee pads (and hand guards), he walked away unfazed and injury-free.

"Protective gear is designed to specially protect you during specific activities. If protective gear exists for your chosen activity, use it."

Once again, protective gear is designed to specially protect you during specific activities. If protective gear exists for your chosen activity, use it. Not all knee injuries can be prevented by the use of protective gear, but many can.

Prevention of internal knee damage, such as ligament and cartilage tears, is discussed in Chapter 11.

SHINS

Nothing beats a kick in the shins to get your attention. It might not be obvious, but football and hockey players wear shin protection under their clothing, as do soccer and baseball players.

Shin Guards

Shin guards can range from thin and strong form-fitting cushions to bulkier hard shells. They prevent cuts and bruises, and are more than worth their weight in protection.

ANKLES

Some people are more prone to sprains than others. Ankles are perhaps the most commonly sprained of all joints. Unless proper rehabilitation is performed, once you have sprained an ankle a few times, it is increasingly likely that you will do so again. As the ankle becomes less stable due to over-stretching of the ligaments, sprains become progressively more severe and can eventually progress to partial and even full dislocations. See Chapter 14 for a full discussion of preventing ankle injury and rehabilitating the ankle after sprains.

Ankle Support

Until one has done their homework and corrected mechanical ankle dysfunction, proper support of the ankle joint is a prerequisite to any activity with ankle sprain potential. There are various elastic anklet socks that may help minimally, but taping provides the most thorough protection. Over the years, many reliable techniques for taping the ankle have been created. We will discuss some of the major ones later in this chapter.

PRIVATE PARTS

Some parts of the body are especially sensitive and uncomfortable when even slightly injured. Protect your "private" parts with available athletic gear; there's no need to let these areas be vulnerable to injury during athletic endeavors.

Men

Nipple Protection

For most runners, the difference between ending a run comfortably and ending it with chafed or even bleeding nipples is the difference between running in a soft microfiber shirt that prevents chafing (or no shirt at all) and running in a generic cotton teeshirt. Other protective options include lubrication and/or adhesive bandages.

Wear a Cup or Jock Strap—You'll Be Glad You Did

If your game involves a ball, physical contact, or even the remote chance of being hit, wear a metal or plastic cup. For other sports, a jock strap will reduce your likelihood of injury to this delicate area.

Women

Sports Bras

Sports bras can provide stability, protection (if padded), safety, and compactness in sports performance. Women will likely want to wear sports bras for any high-impact activities that incorporate significant dynamic movement (such as running), or that require jumping or sudden changes in direction (such as basketball, volleyball, or soccer).

Smooth and flowing activities such as certain types of yoga, swimming, dancing, and cycling are some of the possible exceptions. Sports bras come in many variations.

Women with more muscular upper bodies often prefer the wider straps of traditional double-strap designs to the T-back or Y-back of racerback designs. Well-endowed women have often found that wearing two sports bras, one over the other, gives them the best support, although there are more sports bras being offered nowadays that provide excellent coverage and support for larger-chested women. Sports bras are meant to be tight-fitting to give the best support, but for healthy circulation they should be removed once sports participation is done.

Pelvic Shields

Women are playing all sports in greater numbers, and in high-impact sports such as softball, baseball, and hockey, they may want to consider wearing a pelvic shield or protector, which is usually designed as a removable hard shell or padding attached to sport briefs designed for the female physique.

PROTECTION FOR OTHER BODY PARTS

Wear the gear that is common to your sport. If the correct equipment or padding does not exist to meet your needs, it is worth creating your own. This method has led to the development of much of today's most effective protective gear. There is perhaps no end to the variety of pads created for sports pursuits. Heel "donut" pads, shin pads, chin straps on helmets, hand guards worn by gymnasts, and many other types of protective gear were jury-rigged out of necessity long before they were mass produced.

Gear Needs to Fit Properly

In order for gear and pads to be comfortable and to work correctly, they must fit properly. Make sure that your pads are the right size and that they are well secured. If they slip or slide, they won't provide the protection they should, and they can even cause injury.

"Remember that the other guy is wearing protective gear, too, and is equally willing to hit you as hard as humanly possible, which very well might be harder than anything you have ever felt in your life."

NO ONE IS IMMUNE TO INJURY

A special feeling can overcome us when we strap on protective gear. We may feel untouchable, even invincible, as though we are no longer vulnerable to injury. In fact, nothing could be further from the truth. Remember that the other guy is wearing protective gear, too, and is equally willing to hit you as hard as is humanly possible, which very well might be harder than anything you have ever felt in your life.

Watch an American football game for living proof of the high injury rate that happens even while all the players are wearing redundant protective gear. Respect your own mortality, even when wearing gear, and you'll have a much greater chance of leaving the playing field injury-free.

DEVICES FOR SUPPORT AND STABILITY

TAPE

Trainers have been taping athletes for many decades. Used properly, a roll of athletic tape is worth its weight in gold; it may be responsible for preventing more injuries than any other type of equipment. Tape can provide protection by increasing stability, managing swelling, covering sensitive skin that may be cut or blistered, or by mending or holding other protective gear in place, such as a broken chin strap on a helmet.

A good tape job provides almost absolute protection to the joint or parts in question. Becoming familiar with the many uses of tape is a worthwhile pursuit for anyone intending to follow a physically active lifestyle.

Types of Tape

Structural (Supportive) Taping

The point of structural taping is to provide absolute stability. Trainers have been taping athletes for many decades. They have refined the skill until it has become a fine art. A good tape job provides almost absolute protection to the joint or parts in question. It is a thing of beauty to behold: while it is being applied, when it is finished, and in the exquisite degree to which it protects.

Tape can be applied effectively in a layer that is thinner than your skin and still do a great job, such as with a simple "J wrap" of the ankle. It can also be used in thick multiple layers to make a "Louisiana wrap" on the ankle, or in the way a fighter wraps it on his hands. Becoming familiar with the many uses of tape is a worthwhile pursuit for anyone intending to follow a physically active lifestyle.

An ankle taped in this fashion cannot be sprained because the range of movement is restricted. Structural taping adds support to the body's ligaments and tendons by sharing the load with them. There is a continuum that exists between taping styles. Sometimes it is difficult to name the style that is being used, but the distinction is usually unimportant as long as the tape provides the intended structural support.

Functional Taping

Functional taping is a relatively new style of taping. Rather than providing near-rigid support, functional taping allows for limited range of movement in certain directions while restricting it in others. Functional taping is the "high art" of the tape job. Its flexibility and wide variety of applications make the talented trainer invaluable. Classes in functional taping are available. Ask an athletic trainer, physiotherapist, or sports coach for details.

Preventive Taping

Unlike structural and functional taping, preventive taping is not a style of application, but is so-called because it is used to prevent new injury or reinjury. Preventive tape jobs can be done in structural or functional styles, or simply to add a layer of protection to the skin. If you were concerned strictly with preventing blisters, for instance, you might just cover the part in question with tape.

ORTHOPEDIC SUPPORT

A wide variety of support products are available today that make physical activity more comfortable, more effective, and in some cases possible where it otherwise would not have been. These products may be either generic or custom-made. In both cases, designers are constantly developing new products to better meet people's mobility needs and demands.

Orthotics

Orthotics are support devices designed to correct poor mechanical action or support weakness, usually of a joint, but also including muscles and ligaments. The supports allow for improved function where it would be dangerous at best and impossible at worst for some people to participate in physical activity. Often they are used to create an efficient interface between the user and the outside world.

For example, orthotics for shoes are available that, at least theoretically, correct the footfall, improve the gait, enhance balance, and make movement more correct in every way. Custom orthotics in shoes have been known to greatly improve all aspects of performance, from balance and speed to strength and endurance.

Orthotics can also be designed for the mouth to correct the bite, to make for optimal temporomandibular joint (TMJ) function, and to prevent grinding of the teeth.

When the body is functioning correctly, it can handle greater intensities of high-stress mechanics while working much more efficiently. The net result is reduction in injury coupled with improvements in performance. It's possible to progress through a series of supports as joint function and stability improves. Ever-evolving technology and an ever-increasing understanding of human dynamics are being paired to create remarkably effective orthotics that are also reasonably comfortable.

There are two types of orthotics available, generic and custom-made.

Generic

Generic orthotics are sold over the counter. They are usually quite inexpensive, and designed to meet the needs of the majority of users. Many people find that generic orthotics are quite sufficient for their needs.

Custom

Custom orthotics are usually prescribed and fitted by a professional. They may be prescribed by your physician or physical therapist. Often their cost is ten times or more that of the generic variety. While many people feel that custom orthotics are better, it is not always the case. If a generic orthotic will do the job, as it will for many TMJ problems, there is no need to seek a custom one.

BRACES

Braces are support devices that encourage specific mechanical actions while discouraging others. They are available for participants in almost every sport, and are often designed to prevent certain errors in movement from occurring. For instance, participants in the game of bowling often unintentionally flex their wrist as they release the ball. This action adds a variable that many bowlers would prefer to eliminate.

Hence, a wrist brace has been designed that stabilizes the wrist and reduces extraneous movement. Golfers also have unique braces available to them, as do participants in many other skills, sports, and games. While it is not considered "bad form" to use these devices to create better consistency in your sport, many people prefer to not use them.

ORTHOTIC CRUTCHES CRIPPLE TOO

When considering the use of orthotics and other support devices, it's worth remembering that these tools often compensate for a weakness in the body that an athlete might be able to overcome with proper strength and flexibility gains, or technique improvement.

A fully-grown adult who has one leg that is shorter than another (a true rarity) may find that a inch-thick shoe insert allows him to run pain-free for the first time in years, a gift which cannot be understated. It's unlikely that any amount of training would fully compensate for his shorter leg by itself.

But generally, modern running shoes and shoe orthotics provide perhaps the most widespread example of corrective devices leading to poorer technique and weakness due to muscle atrophy. Modern running shoes literally discourage the use of proper running form, encouraging instead a heel strike technique. The heel strike is not only a slower running form, it is also less stable for the ankle, while also minimizing the use of the calf muscles. Proper running form utilizes calves aggressively.

Far from the early minimalist running shoes of the 1970s , most shoes on the market today include elements to correct perceived faults in the movement of the foot and cushion it from impact. It's also not at all unusual for average runners to have shoe orthotics suggested to them at their local running store.

Yet studies in the developing world have continuously showed populations wearing thick-soled shoes are far more prone to foot and ankle injuries than those who go barefoot because they lack any shoes at all.

Others investigating the newly-emerging enthusiasm for barefoot and minimalist running have found the adherents compensate for their lack of padding by plantar-flexing the foot on contact with the ground, creating a softer and more mechanically correct landing.

Cushioned running shoes also protect runners from the pain they would experience by running in minimalist footwear with bad form. Unable to land on their heels, minimalist and barefoot runners land mid foot, creating more work for the soft tissue support structures, which increases foot strength and possibly reduces the risk of injury.

Of course, when a lifelong padded-shoe runner goes out and tries to run in minimalist footwear, he may at first overdo it and injure himself due to the atrophied state of his foot and ankle musculature. By building up to longer distances slowly, however, he can likely gradually build up to stronger feet that no longer require assistance to function properly.

Whenever you add a new piece of equipment to your fitness routine, it's worth asking yourself this question: "Is this item protecting me, does it allow me to get away with leaving my weaknesses unaddressed, and is its use actually resulting in poor form and further imbalances?"

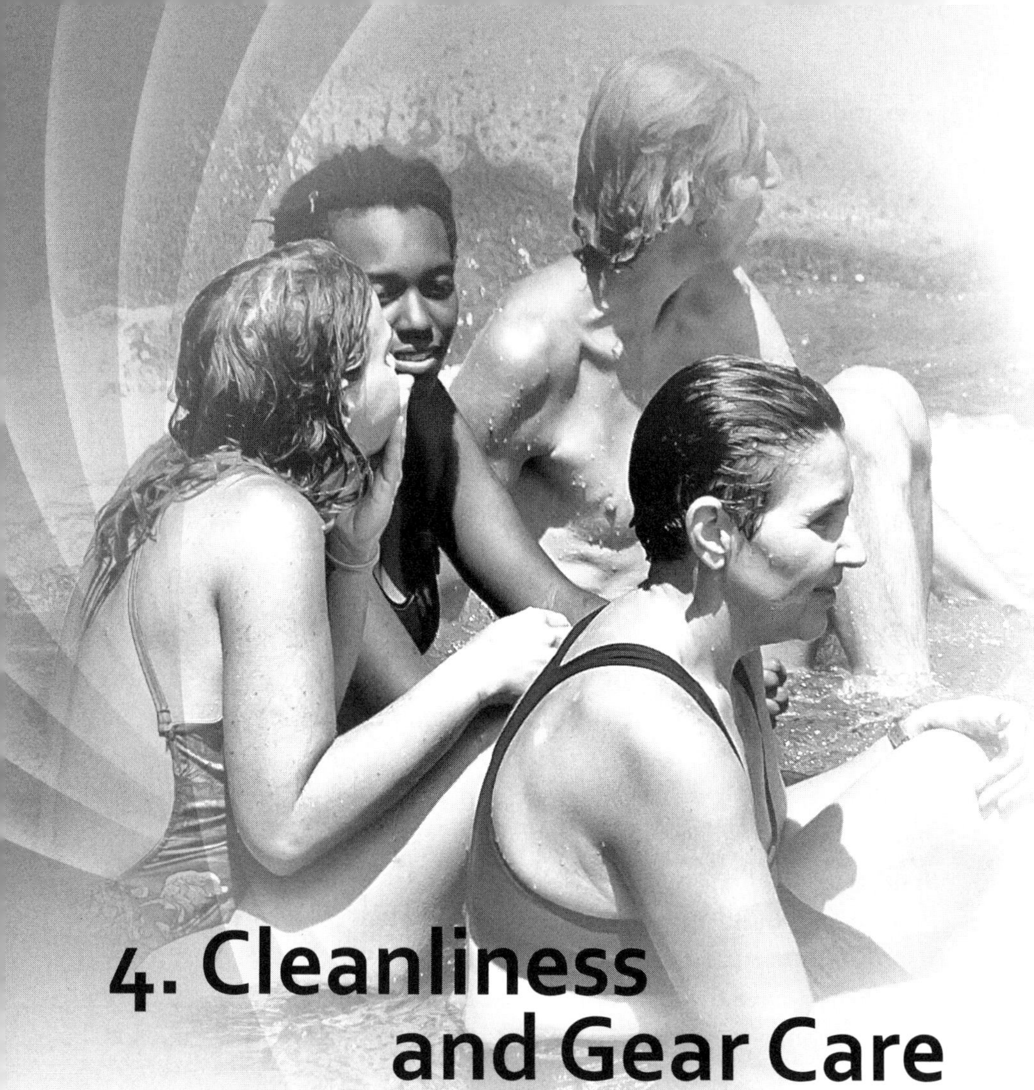

4. Cleanliness and Gear Care

"Cleanliness is next to godliness," or at least so goes the old adage. When it comes to prevention and care of injuries, cleanliness is absolutely vital. Without proper hygiene, we are prone to unnecessary problems and pain when participating in physical activities, and improper cleansing of wounds can lead to infections, slowed healing, and often, severe complications.

Some sports gear is designed to come into contact with our skin. If the skin is irritated, it can make participation in sport uncomfortable and even intolerable. Even our fitness equipment lasts longer and functions better when it is kept clean.

SKIN DEEP

Many factors contribute to the health of the skin. While some of these may seem like common sense, it is likely that some will come as a surprise.

"Human skin requires exposure to sunlight in order to stay clean."

ULTRAVIOLET RAYS ARE THE ULTIMATE CLEANSER OF THE SKIN AND BLOOD

The kidneys and liver function to cleanse the blood, but they are not alone in performing this task. Regular exposure to sunlight also is essential for maintaining clean blood. The ultraviolet (UV) rays of the sun actually penetrate human skin and disinfect the blood while it is within the capillaries. UV exposure is so essential to our health that dialysis machines are designed to expose blood to ultraviolet light for those who are bedridden. For the body to be truly clean it is critical for the blood to be clean—sun exposure is essential in keeping it so.

Human skin also requires exposure to sunlight in order to stay clean. Often the parts of our bodies that have the least exposure to sunlight also have the most objectionable odors, but just a few minutes of direct sunlight will eliminate persistent odors from any exterior part of the body.

CHAFING FROM UNCLEAN GEAR IS HAZARDOUS

Just a few grains of sand rubbing against the skin are an extreme irritant, and a tiny pebble in one's shoe can be disabling. Cleaning your gear thoroughly will help prevent these annoyances from turning into accidents or injuries.

Protective sports gear is often designed to guard our skin, but if the gear is dirty, wet, worn-out, poorly fitting, or otherwise inappropriate, it can make participation in sport painful and even dangerous. A little "no worries" blister can quickly expand to cover a large surface area in practically no time when subjected to the high-stress mechanics of sport. As a rule, the larger the surface area, the longer the time required for healing. Any injury that can be avoided should be avoided. Keep your gear impressively clean.

Sweat Not Washed Away Will Irritate the Skin

The primary component of our sweat—water—evaporates or drips to the ground when we perspire, leaving the solids of sodium and sodium chloride on our skin or in our clothing. These solids form crystalline structures sharp enough to cause abrasions of the skin. Long-distance runners are often rubbed raw from the dried perspiration that accumulates on their clothing.

Whenever possible, rinse with water immediately after engaging in activities in which you perspire. Irritations of the skin are uncomfortable, tend to last longer than we would like, and can lead to more severe conditions.

INFECTIONS

Infections are one of the most common ailments in sport. A serious infection can lead to lengthy periods of little or no training, and can even alter your life permanently. While they can have deadly complications and should not be ignored, infections are relatively easy to avoid by utilizing basic hygiene considerations. All injuries should be washed as soon as possible. Clean water is usually sufficient to clean most wounds. And following sweaty exercise, rinsing oneself in water followed by drying off effectively will help keep the skin in prime condition.

Fungal Infections

Athletes commonly encounter and are susceptible to symptoms caused by microscopic fungus that flourish in warm, moist conditions. Tinea, or “ringworm” (not actually a worm), goes by jock itch, athlete’s foot, and so on, depending on the part of the body where it shows up. It can cause severe itching and scaly patches. By giving sufficient attention to cleanliness (bathing as needed, fresh workout clothes for each session, not sharing towels or clothing) and keeping your skin dry, you will have gone a long way toward preventing fungal skin infection.

Avoiding Jungle Rot

The severe itch that often follows insufficient attention to cleanliness of the feet or crotch always brings repentance. These issues never heal as quickly as we would like, either. Commonly, even after doing the "right thing" and improving personal hygiene, the itch will likely continue for several weeks. When you are involved with sport, prevention of such a malady is far better than treatment. The sheer distraction that comes with even minor fungal skin infections adds unnecessary danger to all other aspects of performance.

Should you find yourself with such an infection, there are many topical lotions available for use without a prescription. Sun exposure can help with the healing, as can diet (see Chapter 8 for nutrition tips), but it still takes time. Infections can become more than a nuisance, as it's not uncommon for people to scratch themselves until their skin is raw, thus complicating the problem by opening the skin to bacterial infection.

Bacterial Infections

Bacterial infections are more likely when a person's vitality has been worn down by poor diet and lifestyle, or they 're in a dirty, poorly ventilated environment that's not exposed to sunlight.

While antibiotics may be used as a last resort when infection has set in, taking them with any regularity can greatly reduce their efficacy and compromise your overall health.

Most Infections Are Self-Limiting

Many people assume that when they see redness around a wound, it means there is infection. This is not entirely true, and it's within the realm of "normal" for there to be a slight reddening of the area around a wound for a few days after an accident. The content of the cells that have actually been damaged must be dealt with by the body, as must the actual cell membranes themselves.

A great deal of anabolic and catabolic activity must be focused on the injured area. The resulting increase in blood flow to the area becomes apparent as redness. If the redness is accompanied by swelling, tenderness, or the area feels hot to the touch, there is likely some degree of infection.

Deeper Infections Can Be Dangerous

Punctures and other deep wounds that do not bleed are especially difficult to clean and are prone to infection. These should be watched closely. Should signs of infection last for more than a few days, you should seek medical attention.

Often, as an injury bleeds, the blood itself carries out any and all contaminants. The lymph that drains from a wound during the first few days after an injury occurs is also a body-generated method of eliminating toxins from within. Traditionally, wounds heal from the inside out. Stitching cuts closed is the common medical practice, which closes them from the outside. This effectively traps anything still inside the wound, such as debris or toxic microbes, increasing the risk of infection. Though your cuts may heal more slowly from the inside out, and might leave a larger scar, they will reliably heal more healthfully in this fashion.

Most injuries heal perfectly, all by themselves. Still, it is wise to be cautious, especially if an injury is deep, covers a large surface area, or damage has been done to the bone. Watch closely for signs of infection, and monitor them should they appear. If the infection around an injury looks serious enough to concern you, seek medical attention.

GEAR CARE

Usually, we don't realize how much we rely upon our gear until it fails us in some fashion. While we may expect athletic equipment to work perfectly every time, indefinitely, the fact is that it just doesn't. Sometimes, when a part of your equipment gives way, it simply creates an inconvenience, such as when the head of a golf club becomes loose, a tennis racket head snaps, a shoelace becomes untied, or a bicycle tire goes flat. There are many times, however, when gear failure can result in serious injury. Once when snow skiing, a critical screw that maintained compression between my boot and binding broke. I was pitched headlong into the woods over a twenty-foot embankment. My airborne momentum was finally stopped when I hit a large tree. Luckily, my injuries were minor.

Another time, I was bicycling with a friend one summer day. We were testing his newest purchase, an amazing bike, indeed. We were far from home, going thirty miles per hour or more down a steep hill when his front rim broke apart. Several hours later, he was released from the hospital full of bruises, stitches, and countless large and small abrasions.

These examples—and no doubt you have a few of your own—show that often, gear failure comes suddenly and unexpectedly, and there is very little we can do about it. On the other hand, broken gear that results from a lack of good maintenance can be prevented. Factors in equipment failure include excessive wear caused by environmental factors, or just plain overuse.

Ultraviolet Deterioration

Long-term ultraviolet radiation from the sun can cause many types of fitness gear to deteriorate profoundly. While you might think that sports equipment is designed to handle these rays, it's best not to count on it. Stitching seems especially vulnerable to solar radiation, such as that maintaining the integrity of your sails, gloves, trampoline, or parachute.

Unless you are certain that your equipment is designed to be left outdoors year-round, it is a good idea to bring it inside after each use. Latex is especially vulnerable to damage from the sun. Products such as resistance bands, inflatable balls (especially large exercise balls), and any products that incorporate latex in their construction are best kept indoors as much as possible to maintain their dependability.

Salt and Chemical Deterioration

To ensure that you remove salt and other contaminants, wash your gear with fresh water after it has been used in the sea, or if you have sweated in it. Equipment that has been used in highly chemicalized indoor or outdoor pools should also be rinsed with fresh water.

Check Athletic Gear Before Use as you would Check Your Parachute

Prior to each use, check to make sure your gear is working properly. Neither you nor anyone else needs to suffer from the delay,

"On any given day, you are essentially betting your well-being on the equipment that you will be using."

inconvenience, and/or injury that you will experience should you suffer an equipment failure. Everything needs to be checked: buckles, straps, moving parts, connections, handles, chains, etc. The axiom "if it can break, it will break, and it will break at the most inopportune time" just might have been coined with sports equipment in mind.

Checking that everything is in tip-top condition is important not just because it is inconvenient when equipment fails. The risk of injury from poorly maintained equipment rises dramatically compared with that from properly kept gear. I have seen people fall straight through trampoline beds that were not replaced in a timely manner, as well as poorly maintained parallel bars that snap, overused sneakers that come apart at the seams during running races, and many other pieces of apparatus fail because they were improperly set up or not given a pre-use check.

On any given day, you are essentially betting your well-being on the equipment that you will be using. If all your equipment is checked and tested as thoroughly as you would check your parachute before jumping out of an airplane, the chance of malfunctioning-equipment related injuries should be reduced to almost nil.

Clean and Maintain Gear after Each Use

After an invigorating and fun activity session, it is tempting to relax. But by cleaning and maintaining your gear immediately after using it, the details will still be fresh in your mind. If you wait until the next time you want to use your gear, you may not remember exactly what part or parts needed attention (it may have been a year or more since the last time you touched that equipment, after all), and you may not have the time to perform the required repairs beforehand. Wash, oil, tighten, retie, and replace as needed, following your workout sessions—you'll thank yourself later.

Planning to take time for gear maintenance as part of your pre- and post-workout schedule will make it easy for you to keep your equipment in top-notch condition and will likely spare you from injury and save you time and money in the long run.

PART 2—Injuries: Failure at the Weakest Link

There is much more to prevention and care of injuries than just exercise and medicine. The health, vitality, and awareness level of each individual plays a vital part in every aspect of injury prevention and recovery.

When any aspect of health is out of balance, the whole is weaker. You can make the most progress with the least amount of effort by attending to your weakest link. By strengthening your weakest fitness link, you will improve your overall health and your training will evolve faster.

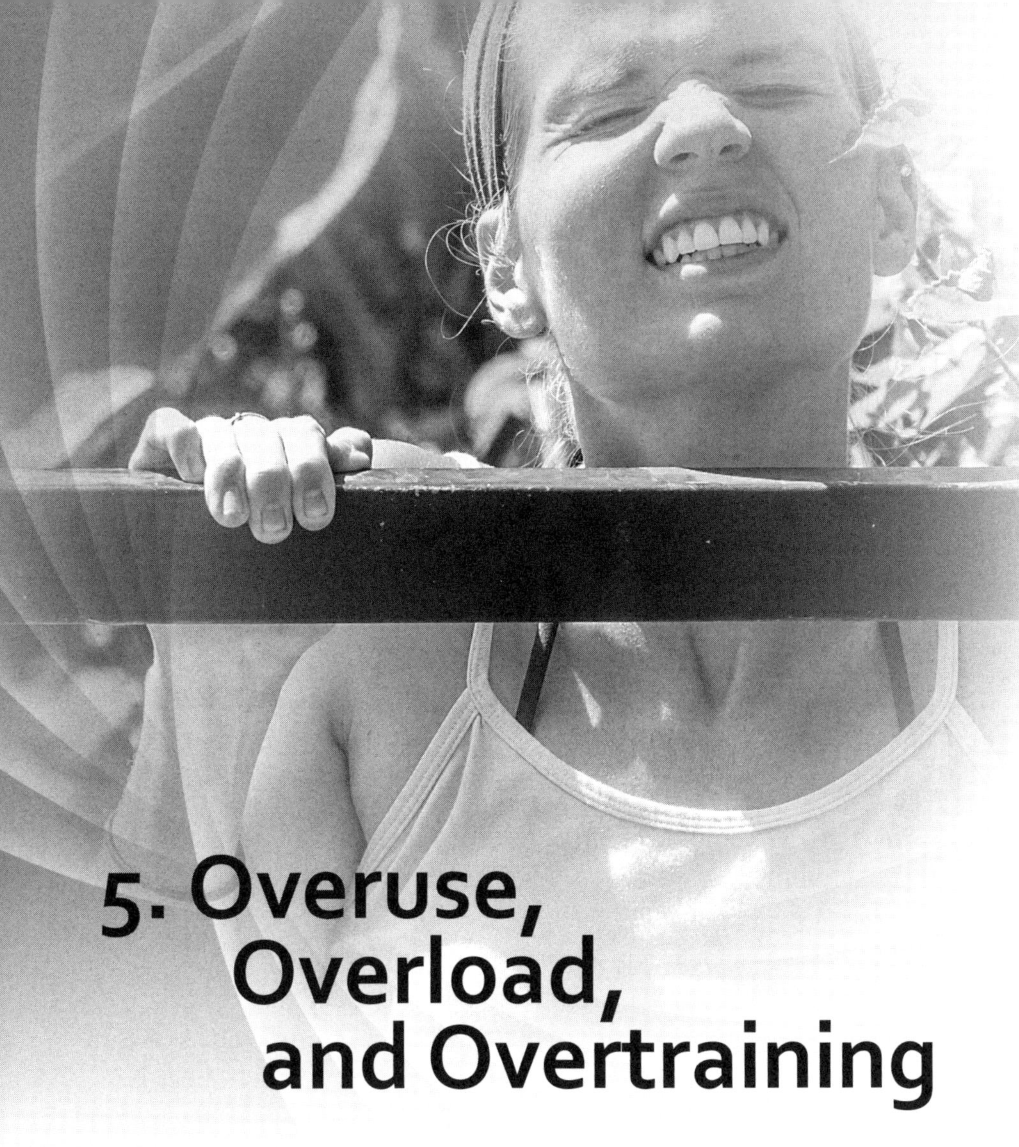

5. Overuse, Overload, and Overtraining

Most of us are more willing to put time and energy into training than we are into recovery. Athletes do themselves a disservice in this case. In an hour or two, we can exert ourselves so severely that it takes days to fully recover. Fully recovered athletes are far less prone to injury because their reaction time, muscle function, and related tissues and systems are in better form.

Understanding the makeup of overload and the warning signs of overtraining will serve to greatly reduce your chance of injury. And appreciating the expected recovery times for overuse and overload injury will help to reduce your downtime.

Defining Overuse, Overload, and Overtraining

Overuse: Using a body part for its designed function but doing so in excess of the part's ability to maintain structural or functional integrity.

Overload: Giving the body a feasible physical challenge that will result in a training effect, an increase in strength, endurance, or neurological skills brought about by the effort.

Overtraining: Placing an unreasonable performance expectation upon any structure or function of the body in terms of intensity, frequency, or duration.

SIGNS AND SYMPTOMS OF OVERUSE AND OVERTRAINING

There is a continuum between the extremes of being perfectly recovered and completely unrecovered. We all fit somewhere within that continuum at all times. At acceptable levels, our degree of recovery leaves us feeling healthy and free of symptoms. However, as the degree of overuse, overload, and overtraining accumulates, symptoms become increasingly overt and eventually, disabling.

Signs and symptoms are actually technical terms with specific and distinct meanings. *Signs* are conditions that can be measured and monitored objectively—such as pulse, respiration rate, blood pressure, and temperature.

Symptoms are subjective: only the person experiencing them is aware of their existence and there is not a way to easily discern or monitor them. Pain, achiness, stiffness, tiredness, or any other vague feeling of discomfort would be classified as a symptom rather than a sign.

"There is a continuum between the extremes of being perfectly recovered and completely unrecovered. We all fit somewhere within that continuum at all times."

WARNING SYMPTOMS

In one study, skiers who practice 32 weeks out of the year tend to ski far better than those who stick to the usual 22. Those who ski 42 weeks out of the year do better still. It was assumed that the group of skiers who tested themselves by skiing 52 weeks of the year would become the best ever.

But the group that skied 52 weeks per year did not do as well as expected, and often did far worse than the others. They were injury-prone, lost their competitiveness, and often even lost interest in skiing. Though they were fully recovering physically, they were not recovering mentally.

Skiing stopped being fun when they had to do it 52 weeks out of the year. Training had become too much like work instead of play, and we all know that while we are willing to play intensely, we tend to become rather methodical about our work, including our work-outs, which can wear us out mentally.

Apathy and Aversion

The joy of movement is a universal human experience, and to be apathetic toward fitness activities is a symptom of poor health. Since there are many lifestyle factors that can adversely affect your recovery, it is actually possible to have the symptoms of being overtrained without having done any physical activity at all. In this case, you are simply underrecovered from lifestyle habits.

Lifestyle factors such as lack of sleep and being undernourished can adversely affect your recovery (and thus your desire to be physically active). However, for those used to an active and healthy lifestyle, apathy toward exercise is one of the first clues that you might be overtraining.

Aversion is a stronger feeling than apathy. By the time overtraining has progressed to the level of aversion, the thought of further training seems almost repellent.

If you have been following an exercise routine for a period of time and are finding yourself not wanting to continue due to apathy or aversion, you are likely overtraining or underrecovering. Reducing the frequency, intensity, or duration of your training will help, as would simply taking a day or two of deserved rest. Chances are that a day of rest will leave you feeling refreshed, excited, and ready to begin your fitness program anew.

Dread of Exercise

You can overtrain to such a degree that you actually come to dread training. As soon as you become aware of such an emotion, take time off from training. If the body's tissues have not properly recovered from prior exertions, injury is looming on the horizon. It is also mentally exhausting to exercise when you don't really want to, which will only compound the problem. Be patient with your body and realize that sufficient quantities of rest and sleep are integral parts of an effective training program.

Perceived Exertion Does Not Match Actual Exertion

People who exercise regularly are generally able to assess how hard they're exerting themselves at any given time. Runners, for example, can usually tell the pace they are running to the minute. But when a runner has been overtraining, what feels like an 8-minute pace could well be 8:15, 8:30, or even slower.

Perceived exertion is a good gauge of an athlete's overall recovery. When perceived exertion rates do not match actual exertion, it is time to take a rest or back off from training. Recovery is an essential facet of training; rest allows the body to take advantage of the training effect. Use perceived exertion as a signal to know when it's time to rest and as an important tool for avoiding injury.

"When perceived exertion rates do not match actual exertion, it is time to take a rest or back off from training."

Performance Decline

Some people participate in fitness routines that allow them to be extremely objective about their training performance. For instance, a person who lifts weights three times a week would likely know exactly how much weight they could expect to raise on any given lift. Ideally, someone on a weight-lifting program would expect to see progress on a regular basis. If performance steadily declines in terms of weight lifted or number of repetitions, overtraining should be considered as a possible reason. After a break of just a day or two, it is common to find that the training effect has brought about the desired results, and the now fully recovered person can once again lift more, not less.

A Cautionary Inner Voice

There is a fairly reliable voice inside each of us that tells us what is safe and what is not. "Why risk it?" the voice asks. "Don't do that, you will likely get hurt," it warns. Self-preservation is a natural instinct, and the impulses we have toward it should likely be heeded at all times to avoid overtraining and injury.

Of course, for a full life, our self-preservation instincts will be balanced by an inner sense of adventure, wisdom gained from prior experiences, and a desire to explore our limits. Learning the difference between challenging ourselves in healthy ways and extending ourselves beyond safe limits is aided by observing warning signs, as well as symptoms.

WARNING SIGNS

Learning to pay attention to the warning signs of overtraining and oncoming injuries can spare you a great deal of pain, frustration, and heartache. In the 2004 Olympics, hurdler Gail Devers was forced to drop out of her secondary event because of a recent injury, but she still hoped to race in the 100-meter event a few days later. Unfortunately, she was only a few steps into that event when she fell with an injury that was likely severe enough to have ended her running career. Had she listened to the warning signals, such an injury probably would not have happened.

Increased Resting Pulse

The term *resting pulse* has several different meanings. For our purposes, resting pulse refers to the heart rate you measure first thing in the morning, in bed, while still completely at rest. This will likely be your lowest pulse of the day.

Your resting pulse is a good indicator of the degree to which you have recovered from your training. Let's say your normal resting pulse is about 60 most mornings. If you find that your resting pulse steadily rises each morning after a series of hard training sessions, it is a good indicator that you are not sufficiently recovering and are likely overtraining. Try to sleep more or reduce your exercise until your normal resting pulse is reinstated.

Many factors can affect your resting pulse. Though they are not all related directly to physical training, they all reflect your overall recovery and ability to perform physically. Dehydration, insufficient sleep, foods that are toxic or difficult to digest, insufficient carbohydrate consumption, malnutrition, sunburn, and many other factors can raise resting pulse. Keep track of your resting pulse and reduce your likelihood of overtraining and injury by adjusting your hydration, sleep, and other recovery factors as needed.

Nagging, Persistent Pains

Pain isn't something you should ignore, particularly if it's persistent. Pain is your body's way of telling you that something is wrong about the conditions it is receiving. It's up to each of us to correct any aberrant situation as soon as we become aware of it and to reinstate ideal conditions for ourselves.

"Nagging or persistent pains—especially those that occur during physical activity—may indicate overuse or overtraining, and usually suggest that more rest and recovery are needed."

Nagging or persistent pains—especially those that occur during physical activity—may indicate overuse or overtraining, and usually suggest that more rest and recovery are needed. When injuries or aches don't heal as rapidly as you think they should, it is also a good idea to seek professional help, such as from a physical therapist or doctor. Once you know the nature of the problem, you will have a far better idea of how to deal with it and know if continued rest is your best option.

Overuse injuries such as tennis elbow, plantar fascitis, shin splints, and many others will respond well only to rest. We can use drugs and therapies to suppress our awareness of symptoms, but only the body is capable of healing itself. Rest is an extremely underappreciated healing modality. The importance of rest and sleep is discussed in detail in Chapter 7.

TYPICAL RECOVERY TIMES FOR VARIOUS INJURIES

When an injury occurs (and if you are active, invariably one eventually will), it can be comforting to have an idea of how long the body should take to heal. By knowing how much downtime is involved, you can confidently assess your situation and engage yourself in proper application of rehabilitation exercises.

There are basically two types of injuries that can occur, acute and chronic. The type of injury has as much or more impact on your recovery time as does the injury's severity. With that in mind, following is a discussion of the various types of acute and chronic injuries that tend to occur when we make miscalculations in applying overload or when we overuse or overtrain our bodies. (We will discuss assessment of severity for a wide assortment of injuries in Chapter 11.)

ACUTE TRAUMA

Acute injuries tend to happen suddenly and unexpectedly, and are usually one of a kind. They tend to require less time for recovery than chronic injuries and are usually—but not always—less severe than chronic injuries. As the acute phase of *any* injury tends to be short-lived by definition, it is understandable that we tend to think of acute trauma injuries as being less severe and shorter lasting.

The acute injuries of overload (a reasonable challenge that results in a training effect), overwork (an unreasonable challenge that results in injury), overtraining (overload at levels of frequency, intensity, or duration that are beyond the body's ability to recover), and overuse (repetitive overload of a specific muscle or joint that is beyond the body's ability to recover) typically fall into the sprain and strain categories. These injuries primarily represent damage to muscles, tendons, and ligaments.

Discerning the type of injury is not always a straightforward process. An ankle sprain is an acute injury every time it occurs, but if it is oft-repeated, one might also classify ankle sprains as chronic.

Muscular Strains

Each muscle is comprised of many fibers, somewhat akin to the way a rope is made from many strands. Should even one fiber tear, you will sense it and probably feel it. This type of injury is referred to as a strain. Strains tend to occur either in the belly (midsection) of the muscle, or out near its very ends.

Muscles dovetail with tendons (which connect the muscles to bones) at each end of their length. The musculo-tendinous junction, where muscle joins tendon, is prone to incurring strain-type injuries. Strains in the belly of the muscle tend to heal more rapidly than strains at the musculo-tendinous junction.

Sprains

Ligaments cross joints, attaching bones to bones. Sprains are injuries to the ligaments, so all sprain injuries occur around a joint. Sprains are tears in ligaments due to being stretched beyond their limits of pliability. Ligaments are relatively slow to heal compared to tissues that have a richer nerve and blood supply, such as muscles. Perhaps of greater importance is the fact that when the ligament material is torn, it is replaced with fibrous material that is not as pliable. Overall this leads to a loss in the joint's range of movement and an increased risk of future tears unless sufficient attention is given to fully rehabilitating the joint and comprehensive warm-up routines are followed.

Sprain vs. Strain, and Other Injury Evaluations

Evaluating the nature and severity of an injury immediately can be difficult. There are a few guidelines, however, that will provide fairly reliable feedback.

Sprains are ligament injuries and will often involve other structures in and around the joint. As such, after experiencing a sprain, the involved joint will be extremely tender when manually assisted through even the smallest range of motion. Essentially, a sprained joint does not want to be moved or stressed in any way.

Strains represent injuries to the muscle and/or tendon, and not to the joint itself. In the case of a strain near the ankle joint, the person will find that the injury only hurts when muscles are used in order to put the joint into motion. Should you attempt to move the joint manually, it will go through its full range of motion with no pain whatsoever, as long as the muscles remain at rest.

If you are still not sure what type of injury was sustained, the "three-day rule" can be extremely valuable. By taking a three-day break from anything that results in pain to the involved part, you will be able to better assess the injury. Most minor strains will heal within those three days, whereas a sprain will usually take closer to three weeks. Should you sustain an injury for which you have not sought medical attention and that does not heal within three days, you might be in for a longer recovery. If fear, worry, or doubt starts to prevail during your healing process, it is a good idea to seek experienced guidance from your doctor or physical therapist.

CHRONIC TRAUMA AND REPETITIVE STRESS

Chronic trauma conditions can arise as a result of endless scenarios. The common factor among them is the existence of a weak area susceptible to damage by trauma. In addition to discontinuing aggravating behaviors, shoring up our weak areas is integral to

"In order to avoid injury and overuse syndromes, it is important to *gradually* strengthen your weakest links in your chosen physical activity."

creating strong bodies and superb health. The "weakest link" concept is an exceptionally important one to understand and utilize when training for any physical activity. When the weakest link in our training is strengthened, our entire program functions better because our body is that much more stable and solid.

In order to avoid injury and overuse syndromes, it is important to *gradually* strengthen your weakest links in your chosen physical activity. For instance, let's suppose a person takes up the sport of running. Having been a swimmer beforehand, this person has excellent cardio ability. However, the cartilage of the knee joint is likely not prepared for more than a few minutes of running without experiencing more trauma than it is ready for. While the acute inflammatory response following overuse of any body part is healthy and normal and no effort should be made to suppress it, it is wise to learn to rest more as a result of experiencing such trauma. By slowly building up the strength of the knee joints, this runner would most likely avoid incurring chronic trauma from overuse.

Tendonitis

Tennis elbow is a classic example of the repetitive stress injury called tendonitis. When tennis players are pushing the limits of their abilities, it is not uncommon for them to be forced into hitting the ball a bit late, or being overpowered by the competition. On the forehand side, this late or hard hit puts extra stress on the medial ligaments of the elbow near the bump known as the medial epicondyle, resulting in microtrauma.

If repeated sufficiently, even microtrauma can add up to significant problems. In this case, the injury is referred to as medial epicondylitis. The outer layer of bone, known as the periosteum, becomes irritated from the trauma of being repetitively tugged upon by the tendon. The periosteum can actually become slightly lifted off of the adjoining layer of bone, as it does in the condition of the legs known as "shin splints." Such irritations are accompanied by inflammation and subsequently, pain.

Resting the injured part is the best and truly only solution for tendonitis. Many people find the disuse distressing, and try to work through the pain, only to find the soreness increases. In severe cases where the pain has been ignored repeatedly, it can take up to two years or more of rest before tennis elbow fully heals. But when caught early, appropriate rest is effective in healing the trauma after only one or two weeks.

Stress Fractures

Long-distance runners who push their training limits while giving themselves insufficient recovery time are prone to a condition known as stress fractures, typically affecting the bones of the foot, but can affect any of the leg bones, and even the pelvis and low back can be involved.

These light fractures truly are broken bones, and should be treated as such. Stress fractures result from the repetitive heel strikes that the foot takes, especially if training is increased too quickly or without taking sufficient recovery. Bones require time to strengthen, to adapt to the stresses to which they are subjected when running. Stress fractures can also result from "pounding the pavement" with an extremely hard heel strike on a paved surface or from running with shoes that provide inadequate shock absorption, such as racing flats or training shoes whose mid-soles have lost their cushion.

Running style makes a huge difference regarding stress fractures. Traditional running style utilizes a heel strike, a style that promotes a lot of shock. In so-called "barefoot running," (there are a variety of shoe designs utilized in barefoot running, and some runners actually run completely barefoot) a style that is rapidly gaining popularity, there is no heel strike, as runners land on the ball of the foot first, like sprinters do.

Barefoot running requires stronger calf and foot muscles, but is showing great promise in terms of reducing the likelihood of running-related injuries, especially stress fractures. Many people argue, quite convincingly, that barefoot running is mechanically more correct than any other style of running.

Stress fractures come about in much the same way that a sculptor breaks rocks; by repetitively tapping them with a chisel and hammer until they give way along the lines of stress. Bones of the foot experience tremendous trauma during running, and if the bones are not allowed sufficient time to recover, they will weaken from such use. Eventually, cracks can appear in the bones. In the case of stress fractures, rest is the only appropriate action, and is required in order for the bones to heal.

Increasing your levels of health and vitality will dramatically lessen your chance of sustaining an injury, and improve your ability to recover from one that does occur. In addition to maximizing overload and minimizing overtraining and overuse, someone who understands and applies the skills of proper post-recovery exertion is less likely to ever sustain an injury. See the next chapter for techniques on how to strengthen your training program through enhanced recovery.

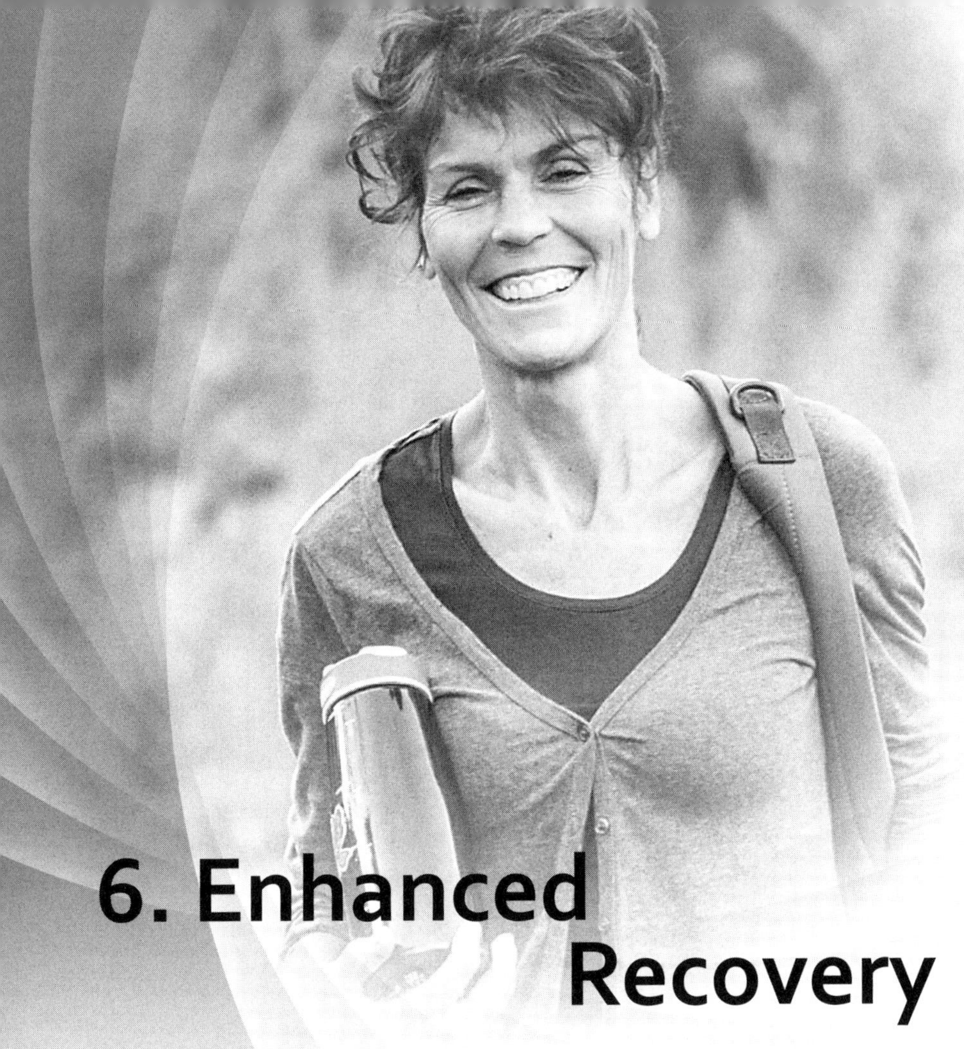

6. Enhanced Recovery

All aspects of physiology are positively affected by the process of recovery. Insufficient time for healing actually holds back physical development and increases the risk of injury. Yet people typically know how to train in far more detail than they know how to recuperate from training. Anyone seeking to improve their athletic performance while decreasing their likelihood of injury needs to place as much emphasis on building their recovery skills, knowledge, and habits as they do on training.

Those who understand and apply proper post-exertion recovery methods will have eliminated a typical weak link in their fitness training. While many of the old rules for recovery are as true as ever, some new approaches provide techniques and technology that remove much of the guesswork about rehabilitation. Recovery has become a science.

STP, RECOVERY OBJECTIFIED

"STP" is a term derived from chemistry and physics that has gained acceptance in a broad number of applications. In its purest sense it stands for "standard conditions of temperature and pressure," but it has grown to be regarded as a situation where as many conditions as possible remain unchanged. When basic external factors can be kept consistent, it is easier to tell the impact of any others upon performance and recovery.

Athletes put their bodies through amazing stresses. Among the many conditions that can slow normal recovery times are insufficient sleep, poor air quality, overconsumption of dietary fat, and underconsumption of fruit. High-level endurance athletes have found that their best performances are when they come closest to achieving a steady state of breathing, fueling, hydrating, and so on. Essentially, they are seeking STP in its broadest interpretation. This discovery has prompted other athletes and coaches to apply the STP principle to their needs, with excellent results. By monitoring heart rate, hydration, rest and sleep, blood sugar, pulse rate, and respiratory rate among other factors, athletes work within tightly controlled parameters that ensure their best performances.

MONITORING AND AIDING RECOVERY: BASIC TOOLS

The basic tools used for monitoring recovery can be used beneficially by anyone. Once you learn the fundamentals and develop the habit of monitoring recovery, it becomes a quick and easy task that only needs to be done occasionally. By keeping track of the various facets of recovery using these basic tools, you will find yourself becoming injured less frequently and recovering more rapidly.

Glucometers, ketone strips, heart rate monitors, and even bedroom clocks and body weight scales have proven to be immensely valuable in evaluating recovery from exertion.

While there are numerous factors that can be monitored in order to track recovery to the nth degree, usually this is not necessary unless you are making your living via physical performance. Following are some of the most fundamental factors you may want to track to determine your degree of recovery.

HEART RATE

Most books on sports performance simply associate recovery with heart rate. As general rule, a well-conditioned athlete's heart rate returns to within 10 percent of normal in less than two minutes. If it takes longer, the workout likely may have been too extreme, or the athlete's level of fitness not commensurate with the intensity of the exercise. Still, there are many more factors that can be monitored in terms of recovery than just resting heart rate.

HYDRATION

Hydration is perhaps the most variable of recovery factors worthy of consideration, and often the most misunderstood. As stated earlier, the weakest link in any aspect of performance is truly the most important, as it is upon this facet that the strength of everything else hinges. When hydration levels drop, our ability to transport nutrients into our cells and to eliminate toxins from them is impaired. This reduction in efficiency of basic cellular functions has a profoundly negative influence upon the body's ability to repair itself and to recover from fitness activities.

Technically speaking, water functions neither as a detoxification agent nor as a cleanser of the body. Water is an excellent solvent, and functions also as a diluter, but it has neither the intelligence nor the ability to cleanse the body. Our bodies cleanse themselves; they direct every aspect of the cleansing process, using water as needed. In fact, the body is perfect in its self-directing capacities in all of its functions. Only the forces, substances, influences, and conditions to which it is subjected can limit the body's health-creating abilities.

"When hydration levels drop, our ability to transport nutrients into our cells and to eliminate toxins from them is impaired."

There are two ways of viewing the hydration/toxicity issue. When a person becomes dehydrated, is their toxin level too high or their water level too low? In fact, both scenarios are often true; toxicity and hydration are related but also separate issues. When a runner perspires heavily and dehydration forces him or her to stop, consuming a few pints of water will usually bring the athlete back to a state of hydration and feeling better. The water in no way detoxified the athlete; he or she simply became more hydrated. The water served to dilute the toxic load within the body to a more physiologically acceptable level that resulted in the athlete feeling better instantly.

Toxicity as a factor in injury prevention and recovery will be discussed in greater detail in Chapter 8. Hydration, injury rates, recovery from injury, and recovery from exertion are each linked to electrolyte levels; another issue that will be discussed in Chapter 8.

Monitoring Hydration

Dehydration makes for very slow sports recovery, as bodily processes are impeded without sufficient water. Overhydration, on the other hand, can lead to excessive loss of electrolytic minerals. Supersaturation of the body's cells due to excessive water intake can make it difficult for the body to proceed with basic functions that rely upon specific mineral concentration levels. Too much water is just as problematic as not enough when trying to achieve the optimal water balance for recovery.

There are four basic techniques for monitoring hydration in order to better achieve STP. One is using a body weight scale both pre- and post-workout to observe the weight of water lost during the fitness session. A second technique is recording the frequency of urination per twenty-four-hour period. Third is monitoring the color of the urine, and fourth is monitoring the volume of urine passed each time.

"Too much water is just as problematic as not enough when trying to achieve the optimal water balance for recovery."

Using a Body Weight Scale

A basic bathroom scale may be the most important tool for monitoring recovery that you will ever use. If you weigh yourself immediately before exercise and again soon after, you will get an accurate insight into how much water was lost. Except for a maximum of a few ounces of fat, all of the weight lost during an exercise session is the result of water loss. This water needs to be replaced—the sooner the better, or recovery is delayed. The nutrients that must find their way into the cells to expedite recovery and the metabolic waste products that must exit the cells are dependent upon an adequate supply of water.

Each pint of water weighs approximately one pound. During a long, hard, and hot fitness session, it's possible to lose as much as six to ten pints of water and possibly more. Seven liters of water weighs 15.4 pounds. It's unsafe to lose more than 5 percent of your body weight during the course of a workout, as that much water loss will put you at serious risk of suffering dehydration, heat prostration, and heat stroke.

This water is best replaced by drinking water, but it can also be replenished via eating plenty of fresh, juicy fruit. If insufficient water is consumed after the training session is completed, dehydration results, making recovery almost impossible. Severe lethargy, weakness, and unexpected but extreme tiredness are often indicators of dehydration. You may not be aware of the degree of your thirst until you start drinking. To ensure optimum hydration and the fastest possible recovery, drink as much water as needed to satisfy your thirst and bring your weight back to its pre-workout level. If you are prone to perspiring heavily when exercising, it is a good idea to drink plenty of water during your fitness sessions as well.

Frequency of Urination

There is some debate about the ideal number of times that a human should urinate during the course of a (24-hour) day. However, it is generally agreed that too-frequent or minimal urination are both signs of ill health or impending ill health.

Too-frequent urination is not only an inconvenience; it is also considered a warning sign of diabetes. Urinating fifteen to twenty or more

"It is generally agreed that too-frequent or minimal urination are both signs of ill health or impending ill health."

times per day is generally considered to be excessive. Whenever a person is urinating this frequently on a regular basis, there is almost certainly an underlying physical problem—or problems—that should be addressed. This one symptom could be related to sugar metabolism, electrolyte balance, kidney function, simple hydration, or some other cause.

Most people in the Western world need to consume more water than they do, and almost all are suffering from some degree of dehydration. A large number of healthcare professionals also agree that urinating less than five times a day represents a serious likelihood of dehydration. Normal and healthy frequency of urination, therefore, ranges between five and fifteen times daily.

From my work with thousands of patients, athletes and nonathletes alike, I have come to recommend eight to twelve times per day as the ideal urinary frequency. This allows a buffer for exceptions without getting into potentially dangerous situations. If you urinate fewer than eight—or more than twelve—times per day, appropriate measures should be taken, beginning with adjusting your water intake.

Color of Urine

The color of the urine can range from almost clear to many shades of yellow, to orange, and even to reddish brown. Urine that is almost clear is considered the ideal color to indicate when a person is healthfully hydrated. With very few exceptions, when urine becomes darker in color, it is a sure sign of dehydration. (One exception is the consumption of certain nutritional supplements in orthomolecular doses—these are extremely high doses, well beyond recommended daily allowances.) The simplest solution is the best one: increase water intake until clarity of urine is restored.

Quantity of Urine

Barring other health conditions such as a bladder infection, the quantity of urine passed at each interval is an excellent indicator of hydration level. When urine volume is scanty, it indicates that copious amounts of water should be consumed until a satisfactory volume is voided.

The body does an exquisite job of recycling water as needed in order to avoid dehydration, and will concentrate the urine in order to do so. When there is a low volume of urinary output, your body is signaling that it has begun conserving water and needs more. Fortunately, passing a low volume of urine is usually something that will catch your attention when it happens. It should not be ignored.

Salinity of Perspiration

Too much sodium is dangerous to humans and leads to dehydration, a performance killer that increases injury rates tremendously by making tissues more brittle. An oversupply of sodium in the body must be diluted to acceptable levels by water so as not to harm the body.

Thus, excessive sodium consumption results in water retention, as the body attempts to dilute the sodium saturated in the cells. Water retention yields poor performance as the ratio of lean mass to total weight and the concentration gradients of other nutrients are adversely affected. Excessive salt consumption also raises blood pressure, which can triple your risk of heart disease and stroke. In quantities greater than necessary, sodium causes us to experience a level of dehydration that can eventually result in death.

Fortunately, we are relatively efficient at eliminating our excess sodium. One of the easiest methods for the body to do so is via perspiration. Salt can be so concentrated in the perspiration that it actually burns the eyes and other delicate tissues. When perspiration dries in your clothing and results in a buildup of salt, the crystals can be extremely irritating to the skin. Athletes have been known to bleed at the nipples when salty clothing chafes them during extended workouts and competitions. There are various preparations sold to prevent such soreness. However, perspiration should not be so salty that it burns the eyes. In fact, it should barely even taste salty. While it is normal for there to be some salt in sweat, the concentration should be low enough so that it does not leave a "salt line" in the clothing.

Most of the sodium we consume comes from salt that has been added to our food. The US national daily average of salt consumption is approximately 5 percent of the lethal dose. If we were not efficient at eliminating the excess through urine and perspiration, it would take less than two months for the accumulation to become deadly.

The intelligent choice is to improve your overall health and athletic performance by reducing salt in your diet now rather than attempting to prevent or treat the symptoms of salt damage later. It is far more effective and health-enhancing to avoid ingesting toxins in the first place than to supplement (in this case, with water) in the hope of negating damage done.

REST AND SLEEP

Sleep is an integral part of our lives and an essential ingredient for health. A deficiency of sleep and rest is so commonplace that most people have come to underestimate its importance. We all know that a loud alarm clock, a cold shower, and a strong cup of coffee won't make up for a good night's sleep.

Yet, as life's obligations increase, many people lose sight of the benefits of getting enough sleep, and most are unaware of its direct relation to injury prevention and recovery. In fact, infants and teenagers, who experience the fastest rates of growth of all humans, require the most sleep. Athletes also typically sleep and rest more than most people. Kenyan runners, for example, known as the best in the world, will commonly spend as much as eighteen hours per day sleeping and lounging.

In order to achieve a steady state of metabolism daily—one that indicates you are fully recovered and ready for the demands of the day—sufficient sleep is a primary requirement. Determining your individual sleep needs and evaluating the quantity and quality of your sleep will be considered further in Chapter 7.

Tracking Sleep

Most people know the general time that they get to sleep and wake up each day; however, by taking note of specific nightly and weekly sleep totals, one can create a useful tool for evaluating recovery. Fewer hours of sleep equates to slower recovery.

"Fewer hours of sleep equates to slower recovery."

Clarity of thought is also directly linked to sufficient sleep, and less sleep increases one's risk of injury due to judgment lapses and slowed reaction time. Simply use your bedroom clock to help you keep track of your sleep totals, and aim for more rather than less sleep.

Bedroom Clock

Your bedroom clock can actually serve a multitude of functions besides simply telling you the time. Learn to use the clock to your advantage and you will have accessed a valuable tool that will rarely, if ever, mislead you. If you are not using a clock to your best advantage, you are missing out on important feedback that can make a huge difference in your recovery while reducing your chances of injury in many ways.

BLOOD SUGAR, FUEL, AND KETONES

We have all had the experience of everything "clicking" for us in an athletic endeavor. In the sports world, we often refer to playing our absolute best as "being in the zone," or "getting out of our head." No matter what we call it, we all wish to duplicate these fantastic performances but are rarely able to. Some athletes will superstitiously wear the same underwear or socks that they wore on their high-performance day, hoping to reproduce those wonderful results. But more often than not, they are disappointed.

Blood-sugar levels have a much greater influence upon sports performance than the socks that you wear or whether you tie your left shoe before putting on your right sock.

Yet very few people other than diabetics ever test their blood sugar. Since sugar is the fuel used by every cell in the body, blood-sugar level gives a good representation of the amount of fuel available to an athlete at any given time. Just as we check the fuel gauge of our car before going out for even a casual drive, we can monitor our personal fuel levels by checking blood sugar. It's amazing to me that anyone—especially pros or aspiring pros—would even consider going out for a fitness activity without doing an in-depth assessment of his or her available fuel levels.

With some methodical testing, it is relatively easy to determine the range of blood sugar at which you perform your best. Usually all that is required to consistently bring your blood-sugar level within your optimal performance range (and keep it there throughout your training session) is some practice and juggling of one's diet.

Keeping blood-sugar levels and other basic physiological parameters within STP will greatly enhance your mental awareness during fitness activities, thus reducing your likelihood of injury. Applying the STP concept will also encourage rapid recovery after fitness sessions while enhancing your recovery from injury.

Glucometers

Glucometers are tools that are used to measure blood-sugar levels. They are primarily used by diabetics in order to make sure that their sugar levels do not go too high. However, for the active individual, the glucometer is also an invaluable tool. A blood sugar reading can signal the appropriate food to eat at any given mealtime: either fruits or vegetables.

For instance, if you have just finished a long training session and are ready to eat, you will often find that blood-sugar levels are slightly lower than average. Fruit would be the best food of choice in this situation. However, if you want to eat again a few hours later but have not moved much in the meantime, you will likely find that your blood-sugar level is completely normal. In this case, there is no advantage to be gained by eating more fruit.

Vegetables supply the fewest calories per bite of all foods and are a rich source of minerals. When blood-sugar levels are normal or higher than normal, it is better to fill up on a meal of vegetables. Their volume will satiate you while your body uses the nutrients to balance blood and body chemistry, all without bringing the blood-sugar level out of its normal, healthy range.

For many meals, a combination of fruits and vegetables is likely most effective. Nutrients that need to be consumed as well as the relevant food-combining issues will be discussed in Chapter 8.

Ketone Strips

Ketone test strips are a simple, over-the-counter tool that can be very helpful in determining your degree of recovery from exercise. Measuring ketone levels can prove extremely valuable, especially in situations where endurance activities are taken to great extremes or where weight loss through calorie restriction is one of the goals of the program.

Ketone test strips are dipped into one's urine and indicate the presence of ketones either through a color change of the absorbent pad or via a numeric value for the amount of ketones found in the urine.

When the body has insufficient sugar to fuel itself, it burns body fat reserves, which produces ketones as a byproduct. Assessing ketone levels can help give a picture of the amount of fat being utilized as fuel by the body.

Ketones have a disorienting impact on human awareness and thus have the potential to be dangerous even at relatively low levels. Monitoring the urine for ketone production helps ensure that sufficient carbohydrates are being consumed and that injuries due to ketone-induced poor judgment are avoided. Low- carbohydrate high-fat diets exacerbate the problem of excess ketone production and are therefore contraindicated for anyone seeking health and fitness.

PULSE RATE

Most people have taken their pulse or had it taken at least a few times in their life. You can find your pulse by applying light pressure from the index and middle fingers to the opposite wrist, about an inch below the pad of the thumb. Feel around gently until you find it. Pulse rate

"If you increase the duration, frequency, or intensity of your training, you will require more sleep to properly recover."

represents heart rate: each throb of the pulse follows a beat of the heart.

In bed, first thing in the morning while still at full rest, you will generally find that your pulse is at its lowest rate of the day. This is a reliable time to check it and compare it to prior days. Get to know your resting pulse rate so that you know how you are recovering. If your morning pulse rate is gradually rising, it is likely that you are not getting sufficient sleep to recover from the stresses of your day.

Whether the stresses are physical, chemical, or emotional, increases in stress call for increases in sleep. If you increase the duration, frequency, or intensity of your training, you will require more sleep to properly recover. Tracking pulse rate is an excellent tool for monitoring the progress of your recovery. If you haven't fully recovered, take this into account when planning your upcoming fitness activities as well as your sleep needs.

RESPIRATION RATE

Your respiration rate tells you a great deal about the degree of effort you are currently expending. It's a good indicator of progress in your recovery, both short- and long-term. When you are out of breath you are obviously not recovered. When you catch your breath, you have recovered to at least to a limited degree. In the same way that your resting pulse signals how well recovered you are, respiratory rate tells you how much recovery is needed.

Until respiratory rate comes all the way down to its slowest resting rate, you are not fully recovered. Respiratory rates are lowest when you are sleeping, indicating that you are doing the least possible amount of work at that time. If you are busy digesting a heavy meal during sleep, more work is being done and your respiratory rate will be proportionally faster. The depth and quality of your sleep will likely also be adversely affected, and your total need for sleep increased.

As in many cases of laboratory and vital signs, "normal" does not necessarily equate with "healthy." The typical resting pulse is around 72 beats per minute, and the average resting respiratory rate is near 16. Healthy rates would be closer to 48 and 8, respectively.

You can't accurately monitor your own respiratory rate, because attempting to do so affects it (generally, when measuring your own, you will tend to slow it down). Someone should measure for you, preferably at a time when you do not know they are doing so.

FOUR STAGES OF RECOVERY

Our ability to recover effectively from training is integral to our overall health. Physical exertion and recovery are interdependent: athletes perform more intensely, more frequently, and for longer periods of time when their recovery is efficient, and they recover more rapidly when they are highly conditioned.

One of the surest signs that an injury is waiting in the wings is slowed recovery. For example, if you typically need two days of rest to feel fully recovered from your strength-training program and then it takes four, it is likely that muscles, tendons, or other connective tissues are being stressed too close to their tearing point.

Recovery is most accurately explained as a continuum, ranging from all-out activity during which almost no recuperation occurs, to deep sleep that provides unequaled healing. We will discuss recovery in terms of four basic stages to show how you can better integrate healing and rest into your training program.

IMMEDIATE

"Immediate" recovery refers to the shortest-term aspects of recovering: Those that happen in the midst of physical exertions. A person performing wind sprints, for example, might run for thirty seconds with a pulse rate of 180 beats per minute, but during one-minute recovery breaks between sprints, the pulse rate would drop below 100. As the runner repeats the process five to ten times, pulse and respiratory rates will come down more slowly after each sprint, meaning that the runner is taking longer to recover.

Immediate recovery also occurs when a runner alternates between relatively fast running and slow jogging, using the jogging time to recover. Recovery is represented in this case simply by the catching of one's breath and the slowing of one's heart rate. These changes signal a step down in exertion rate, often from anaerobic to aerobic, or to a less-demanding aerobic state.

You'll find that most sports have recovery built into them.

During a tennis match, there are several reasons for lulls in the action. Some points require extreme exertions while others are slower and easier. Between points, there is a brief break. Each time the players change sides, there is a longer break.

In basketball, all action stops each time a foul is called, and everyone rests between quarters. The game of soccer is filled with pauses in the action, as is football and most other sports. Every break and slowing down of activity represents a chance for participants to recover to some degree.

All of these variations on the in-game break will not allow for full recovery, however. Only full rest (the cessation of all activity) can supply the best conditions for the fastest immediate recovery.

SHORT-TERM

The next stage of recovery, "short-term," represents every type of recovery that occurs in the time frame between immediate and daily recovery. For example, half-time at most sports games gives the athletes a short-term recovery opportunity. And if you play basketball in the morning and jog in the afternoon, there is plenty of time for short-term recovery in between.

After just a few hours, you probably will not have fully recovered in the specific body parts that were used during the previous activity. Still, general physiological parameters such as pulse and respiration rates will have recovered sufficiently to take on another session of fitness activities even after such a fairly short rest. Pushing the limits of short-term recovery, however, will extend the amount of time needed for complete daily recovery.

DAILY

If you wake up in the morning with the energy and enthusiasm of a five-year-old child, you have likely recovered fully from the prior day's exertions and challenges. If you find that you have a difficult time getting started in the morning, you are likely still unrecovered and would benefit from a day of complete rest. Should you choose to put in another full day of training without allowing for more extensive recuperation, you will lose ground in recovering sufficiently, leading to steady declines in performance and increased risk of injury. Extending yourself in ways that exceed the limit of your ability to recover daily also means injuries will take longer to heal, often naggingly so.

One way to make recovery more efficient is to vary the physical challenge you choose to do from day to day. One option is to choose from the five different classes of activity—muscular strength, muscular endurance, flexibility, neurological, and cardiorespiratory—and train in different ones on different days. For instance, by alternating running and lifting weights on different days, you double the specific recovery time available for each type of exertion.

Another way to achieve the same result is to vary your choice of activity within any specific session. Triathletes, for example, participate in three different types of cardiorespiratory exercise: running, swimming, and bicycling. Often, they will alternate between the three, doing only one or two of the exercises on any given day. Each of these exercises uses different primary muscle groups. Recovery is easier and more rapid for the multisport athlete than it is for the distance runner who might be tempted to train by running long distances day in and day out, using the same muscles each time.

"Recovery for the multisport athlete is easier and more rapid than it is for the distance runner who might be tempted to train by running long distances day in and day out, using the same muscles each time."

Day-to-day recovery is an ongoing process, but progress occurs primarily when we are sleeping. During the day, progress and regress are both happening, and overall there is a net loss. The amount of recovery accomplished each night depends greatly upon the quality and quantity of your sleep. It also relies heavily upon factors such as nutrition, the weather, and mental attitude, which will be discussed in detail in Chapters 8, 12, and 15, respectively.

SEASONAL

One of the advantages of being athletically well-rounded is that a variety of activities can be pursued during different seasons. Recovering from season to season, by resting certain muscle groups while training others, is the very essence of cross-training. This strategy makes year-round activity much more enjoyable and helps to keep one's attitude toward fitness fresh.

Our bodies respond well to varied movements and stressing different muscle groups throughout the year; in fact, the training effect can be minimized when we perform the same movements year-round. For people who are enthusiastic about overall fitness even more than they enjoy participating in one particular sport, taking advantage of the wide assortment of activities available throughout the year makes recovering seasonally easy and effective.

Many people choose to use the colder portion of the year (in temperate climates) or the rainier or hotter part of the year (in the tropics and subtropics) to concentrate on aspects of fitness which they neglect during the other parts of the year. Many of these are done indoors in gyms or houses, where the weather isn't a factor.

Others are influenced by the seasonality of their chosen sport.

Regardless of how weather patterns and event calendars influence your year, you may want to occasionally pick a few items off the following chart to work on aspects of your fitness you don't normally address.

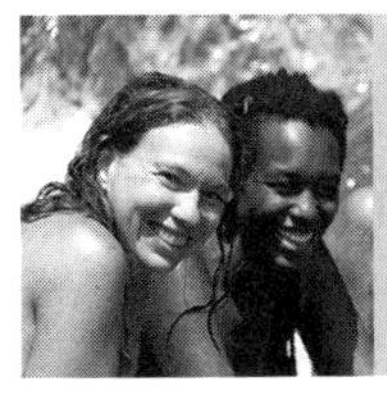

- Swimming in an indoor or outdoor pool, lake, or ocean

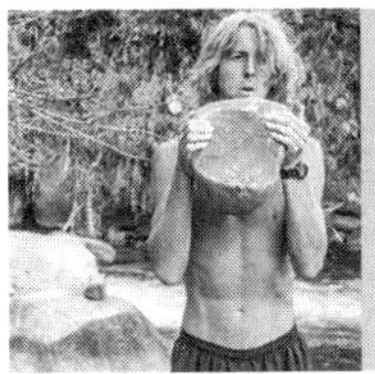

- Lifting heavy rocks, logs, or barbells

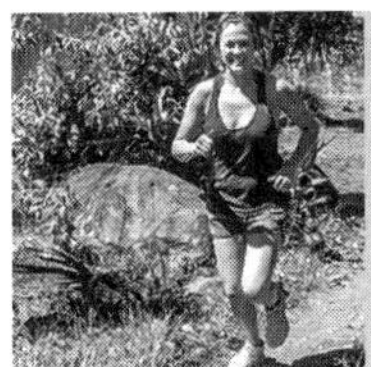

- Sprinting or running long distances on an indoor or outdoor track, road, or treadmill

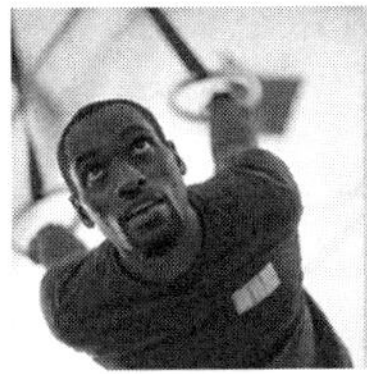

- Gymnastic exercises such as handstands, handstand walking, planches, cartwheels, or ring dips

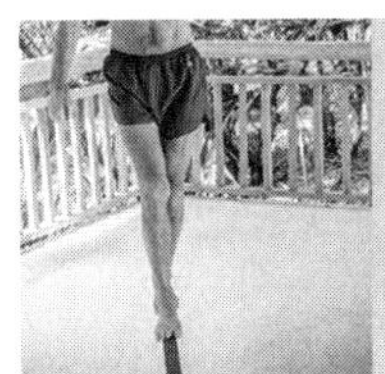

- Balance work on a slackline, wobble board, or tightrope

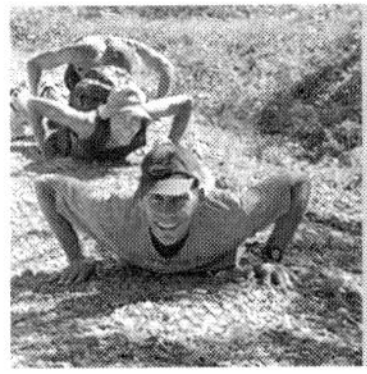

- Bodyweight exercises like pushups, pullups, or squats

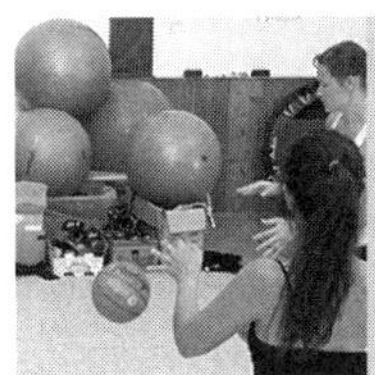

- Juggling

Understanding What Your Body Needs

Knowing when to push and when to rest is an art form for those who are dedicated to fitness. Monitoring your immediate, short-term, daily, and seasonal recovery status helps tremendously in this process. Many people have found that taking as little as a week to as much as a month or even longer to focus on rest and recovery ultimately improves their performance. You are not alone if you find it challenging to take an entire week off from training. But it's important to remember that resting is not "doing nothing"—it's an integral part of training and health to allow the body time to go into "active healing" mode. Rest is an extraordinarily valuable activity that can make the difference between fully recovering and improving performance and overtraining to the point of injury.

UNDERRECOVERING VS. OVERTRAINING

When it comes to injuries, overtraining is usually not the main problem. In fact, underrecovering is responsible for a far greater number of injuries. When we speak of overtraining, it is relative to the amount of time we give to recovery. When we refer to underrecovering, we are including all of the lifestyle factors, conditions, forces, influences, and substances that play a role in our recovery. Sufficient rest and sleep, clean air, pure water, emotional poise, foods appropriate for your specific nutritional needs, adequate daylight and sunlight, plus many other factors, all must be sought if you truly wish to recover optimally. By becoming more adept at participating in all of the forces of recovery, you will be able to pursue your fullest training capacity. For more details on recovery, refer to my book, *Nutrition and Athletic Performance.*

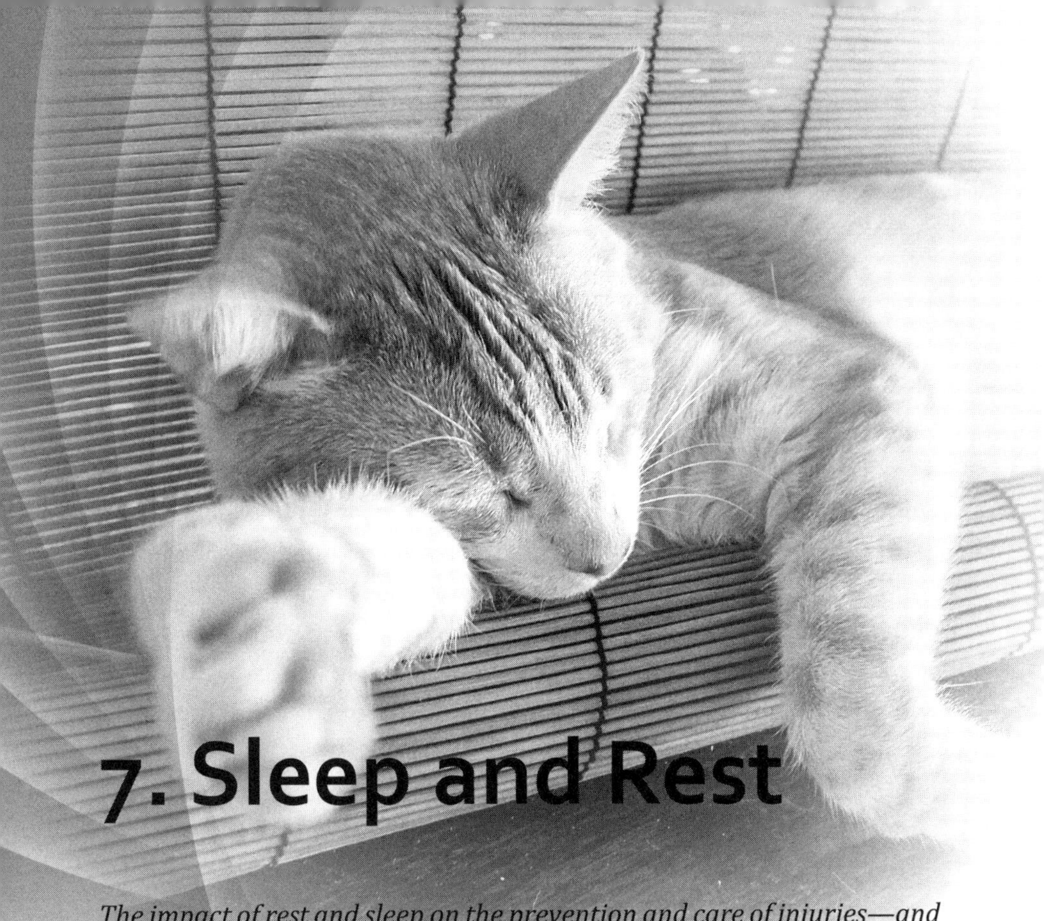

7. Sleep and Rest

The impact of rest and sleep on the prevention and care of injuries—and human health in general—is so great that it deserves its own chapter. In fact, I would not be surprised to see entire books dedicated to the importance of rest and sleep on human performance in the future. Do not let this invaluable aspect of training become your weakest link.

Many people consider a good night's sleep a luxury; however, sleeping fully and deeply at night on a regular basis is truly a necessity for consistent health on all levels. Almost everyone would benefit greatly by increasing the quantity and quality of their rest and sleep. The underslept person is more likely to sustain an injury, as well as take longer to fully recover.

Every level of health hinges on sufficient sleep. Nutrition, fitness, mental attitude, emotional poise, and all detoxification processes function optimally only when we are well-slept.

"The brain produces nerve energy in the form of low-voltage electricity, and then uses it to direct the functioning of every cell and every function of the body."

THE ROLE OF SLEEP

Sleep provides time for the detoxifying functions of your body to outpace the toxifying conditions to which it is exposed on a daily basis. During sleep, anabolic processes (the creation of complex structures from simpler ones) exceed the rate of catabolic ones (the creation of simpler structures from more complex ones). This allows for growth and repair within the body. While the body is asleep, the brain makes sense of the day's input, experiences, and exposures, cataloging and directing the body's functions in order to make the appropriate repairs and adaptations.

Perhaps the most important role of sleep is the accumulation of vitality that we call "nerve energy." The brain produces nerve energy in the form of low-voltage electricity, and then uses it to direct the functioning of every cell and every function of the body. It also takes nerve energy to demonstrate enthusiasm of any kind, and to exert ourselves in any manner.

Nerve energy is produced by the brain twenty-four hours a day, every day. When we are awake, we use this energy more rapidly than it can be produced. Thus, when our supply of nerve energy runs low, we feel the urge to sleep. When we feel tired we have usually not completely run out of nerve energy, but have run low enough that the body requires sleep to recharge itself.

In case of emergency, some nerve energy is usually kept in reserve. However, we drain these reserves when we use an alarm clock to jolt us awake, consume stimulating foods and beverages such as meats and caffeinated drinks, or when we in any way rely upon outside stimulants in order to have a sense of being "energized."

When we are asleep, we produce nerve energy faster than it is being used. In this way, we accumulate nerve energy for use at a higher rate when we are awake, free of external stimulants.

The Sleep Stages: NREM 1, 2, and 3 and REM. When we fall asleep, we progress though a number of phases: non-rapid eye movement (NREM) stages 1 through 3 followed by rapid eye movement (REM), and then we begin again at stage one. In a normal night's sleep, we will go through this cycle about four or five times.

What most people would describe as "dozing" is actually stage 1 sleep, when the brain is experiencing alpha brain waves This is the lightest sleep we experience. Stage 1 typically includes our experience of falling asleep and waking up.

During stage 2, when the brain is producing theta brain waves, the body prepares to enter true sleep. The muscles go through spontaneous periods of contraction mixed with muscle relaxation. The heart rate slows and the body temperature decreases.

In the even deeper sleep of stage 3, when the brain is producing delta brain waves there is a larger decline in heart rate and blood pressure accompanied by a relaxation of the musculature. If you are awakened from stage 3 sleep, you may find it almost impossible to move or think coherently. The expression "like trying to wake the dead" aptly describes trying to awaken someone from stage 3 sleep.

Most dreaming occurs during REM (rapid eye movement) sleep. Sometimes, muscle twitches accompany or slightly precede dreams as well. It's different from non-REM sleep as heart, blood pressure, and breathing become irregular. A drop in body temperature accompanies REM sleep.

We spend a different amount of time in each stage of sleep, yet scientists have proven repeatedly that each of them is required for health.

TIPS FOR SLEEP QUANTITY AND QUALITY

QUANTITY OF SLEEP

How much sleep do you need? Enough. Anything less than enough is not enough. How can you tell if you have had enough sleep? When you want to roll out of bed and start your day rather than roll over and go back to sleep, for starters. Sleeping until you feel fully refreshed is always the best option.

A body builder came to me once asking why she wasn't getting the results she wanted and expected. She was training diligently yet was not gaining muscle size or losing body fat. After taking a comprehensive history, my suggestion to her was simple. "Your diet is impeccable. Your training is perfect. You simply aren't getting enough hours of sleep. Six hours of sleep is not enough for you to grow. Add three hours of sleep to your program every night for a month." She argued for a while that she was getting all of the sleep she needed, but eventually she decided to take my suggestion, as nothing else that she had tried had worked.

The results were incredible. She started dropping fat and gaining muscle. Before the month was over, she increased her sleep to ten hours per night and committed to another two months of the "experiment." Her growth became truly fantastic. Her trainers couldn't believe their eyes and wanted to know the name of the "miracle drug" she was using. She told them it was called "sleep," and that they ought to try it. She gained three inches of muscle in her biceps and calves, and four inches of muscle in her thighs and chest. She lost over eighteen pounds of fat and four inches off her waistline, and gained over twenty pounds of muscle.

Needless to say, she has continued the program to this day, now sleeping eleven hours per night. She is still making astonishing strides in her training, developing strength and size at an unheard-of pace. She now recovers in three days from workouts that used to take ten days for recovery.

Can You Sleep Too Much?

All too often people tell me that they need to limit their sleep because if they allow themselves all the sleep they desire, they will "never get up," and invariably wake up in the morning more tired than they were when they went to sleep the night before. I explain to them that they are only touching the tip of their sleep deprivation. Really, they are just beginning to get in touch with their true tiredness. Many people deprive themselves of necessary sleep by possibly three to six hundred or more hours per year, every year, for most of their lives, so getting a few extra hours in now and then will not make up for the lack. Try to sleep as much as possible, whenever your body has the inclination.

Remember, your body is running its own show. It has its own agenda, which takes priority over yours. Your body is self-directing, self-healing, self-organizing, self-controlling, self-monitoring, and self-repairing. It depends upon you to provide healthful conditions, substances, forces, and influences in order for it to create the optimum health we all desire.

By ignoring sleep debt with the misguided objection that the body will always want more and more sleep, we are thumbing our noses at its attempts to maintain homeostasis. Sleeping too much is not possible. If you do not need sleep, you cannot sleep. If you do need sleep, you are likely to fall asleep even at inappropriate times, such as in movies, lectures, while reading, or when watching television. If you can fall asleep, you need to sleep. In a healthy state, the body cannot oversleep any more than it can overdigest your food or overurinate. When your need for sleep is fulfilled, your body will make that exquisitely clear by producing a state of alert and aware wakefulness.

By providing yourself with sufficient sleep, your body will take care of a great deal of the remaining details required for health without your being consciously aware of them. Daily recovery will be optimized while recovery from injury will proceed as rapidly as possible. The sharpness and clarity that comes with being well-slept greatly reduces your chances of incurring injuries of any type.

The secret to getting sufficient sleep is in getting to bed at a reasonable hour. It takes practice, but eventually you can regain your innate love of, and desire for, being well-slept. Going to bed will become an activity you look forward to because you will associate it with helping create the physical vitality and mental clarity you desire. Being well-rested provides so many rewards

"The secret to getting sufficient sleep is in getting to bed at a reasonable hour."

that staying that way is its own motivation. Once you have tasted the benefits, there will be no turning back.

QUALITY OF SLEEP

Everyone desires a good night's sleep and quality is as important as quantity if we want to sleep deeply and soundly each night. Unfortunately, it is not uncommon for people to experience restless or poor sleep due to stress, diet, and other factors.

Primarily, in order to get a good night's sleep, one must be comfortable. Fresh air should circulate in the sleeping environment. The temperature needs to be just right, neither too hot nor too cold. Irritating sounds or smells should not intrude upon the sleeper's peace. The sleeping surface itself should not be too hard, lumpy, soft—or objectionable in any other way. Total darkness encourages the best sleep. Even the food you eat and when you eat it makes a difference in the overall quality of your sleep.

The Impact of Food on Sleep

For the body to experience deep and restful sleep, energy demands must be minimized. The digestion of heavy, difficult to assimilate, or large quantities of food late in the evening reduces our ability to achieve deep sleep due to digestion's high-energy demand.

Eating in this fashion also seems to greatly increase the likelihood of nightmares. Foods that are particularly difficult to digest include meats, nuts, cheese, and combinations thereof. With the possible exception of a light snack of fresh fruit or vegetables, the best quality sleep is realized when we go to bed after having not eaten for several hours.

Many people use food as a drug, and eat so heavily that they actually seem to fall asleep after a meal. In reality, the digestive demand has become so great that it is no longer possible to maintain consciousness. Essentially, the eater has gone comatose after eating such a meal and, like after any drug overdose, is sleeping it off. We do not accumulate the same benefits of sleep from this "false sleep." You could sleep for two hours after a large holiday dinner for example, and still require a full night's sleep later in the evening.

Any time we eat until unconsciousness results, we are exerting a negative influence on all of the body's systems, including our ability to recover mentally as well as physically. For optimum injury prevention, clear-headedness is an absolute requirement.

Excitotoxins

Excitotoxins are a class of chemicals often added to prepared and packaged foods. They have a stimulating effect on the brain (excito) while also functioning as cell destroyers (toxins) within the brain. The most powerful and common of the excitotoxins are the glutamates, commonly added to food in the form of monosodium glutamate (MSG).

Consumption of MSG or any other excitotoxins results in aberrant brain chemistry—excitotoxins adversely affect the electrical functioning of the brain. The resultant misfiring of the brain's neurons often leads to mental confusion, uncoordinated physical movements, and even behavioral changes.

Because excitotoxins stimulate the brain, they make achieving high-quality or deep levels of sleep impossible. The damaging effect of excitotoxins on sleep and health is far-reaching and cumulative. Anyone wishing to maximize their athletic performance while minimizing recovery time should eliminate the use of all excitotoxic substances. For further reading on excitotoxins, refer to the Bibliography.

SLEEP AND HUMAN PERFORMANCE

There is no bright side to sleep deprivation: it results in lowered yield from physical activity, reduced desire to exercise, decrease in positive mental attitude, and increased risk of injury among other outcomes. Sleep deprivation is so detrimental that it is considered a significant factor in traffic and workplace accidents as well as in sports injuries. Sleep deprivation for twenty-four hours has been shown to have effects comparable to that of a blood-alcohol level of 0.1 percent (legal impairment). Getting all the sleep you desire, on a daily basis, is a critical factor in virtually every aspect of mental and physical functioning and recovery.

"Decision-making, mental focus, concentration, short-term memory, organizational skills, and many other facets of brain activity become unbalanced as sleep deprivation accumulates."

When it comes to sleep's impact on human functioning and performance, it is difficult to separate the physical from the mental because the brain is responsible for all of the body's physiological and mental processes. We cover the functions separately below in a philosophical rather than anatomical sense.

SLEEP AND MENTAL FUNCTIONING

Sufficient sleep is essential for proper mental functioning. Mental clarity is compromised relative to the amount of sleep missed, and it has been suggested that all brain functions are impaired relative to the amount of sleep deprivation one suffers. Decision-making, mental focus, concentration, short-term memory, organizational skills, and many other facets of brain activity become unbalanced as sleep deprivation accumulates.

With loss of mental focus comes an increased propensity for injury. Small errors in judgment can escalate and often result in unnecessary accidents. Sleeping sufficiently is required for mental clarity and will dramatically reduce your chances of injury, as well as aid you in healing from those injuries that do occur.

SLEEP AND PHYSICAL FUNCTIONING

Impaired coordination is somewhat proportional to lost sleep, raising the possibility for injury accordingly. Increased risk of stress fractures, lack of incentive to train, and general tiredness, are all related to sleep deficiency. Insufficient sleep keeps the training effect from fully maturing, and thus reduces the benefits of training.

Sometimes getting a small cut or bruise catches our attention and lets us know we need more sleep or rest, and to be more careful in the meantime. At other times, we may miss the warning signs and symptoms and find ourselves suffering with a severe injury and schedule setback. Getting enough sleep heightens your energy and physical prowess, and helps keep you injury-free.

SLEEP AND RECOVERY

The role of sleep is critical to recovery. Anabolic and catabolic activities are both continuous, ongoing functions; however, anabolic activities have the opportunity to outpace catabolic ones while we sleep. We see how the rapid growth (anabolism) of infants and teens is accompanied by the need for an enormous amount of sleep. During sleep, the body is in a heightened state of growth, healing, and cleansing. The same holds true whenever a training effect is initiated: it should be matched by increases in sleep and rest time, or recovery will be inhibited.

With insufficient recovery, the waste products of cellular metabolism are not fully eliminated from your tissues and nutrient uptake is not completed. These factors have a compromising influence on cellular structural integrity, and make injury more likely. Reduction in recovery rates will also lead to loss of energy and enthusiasm for the day's activities, thus impairing overall training. Furthermore, slowed recovery reduces your ability to heal from exertion and injury.

NAPS

Salvador Dali was famous for taking catnaps. He claimed that all he needed was a very short nap in order to feel revitalized. His system of napping was to place a plate on the floor next to the chair in which he slept. He then placed a small spoon in his hand, which he positioned above the plate. As soon as he fell asleep in this position, the spoon would fall from his hand, hit the plate, and wake him up, fully refreshed (he claimed), from his nap.

In all likelihood, Dali's naps were not long enough to be as rejuvenating as he suggested. As discussed earlier, there are three non-rapid eye movement stages of sleep, prior the beginning of the deep and restorative REM sleep. Each is somewhat deeper than the one before, and it's essential to reach the deeper levels in order to wake truly refreshed from a nap.

WHEN TO TAKE A NAP

Many cultures around the world are proud to take afternoon siestas. Taking a nap should not be an activity for which you feel the need to apologize. The best time to take a nap is any time you feel like sleeping during the day. Many people find themselves remarkably more productive by breaking their day into two halves separated by a nap than by trying to be active all day.

If you can sleep, you likely need sleep. Instead of fighting the urge to sleep by reaching for stimulating foods, drinking coffee, listening to music, or exercising during the day, a healthier move would be to get some sleep in the form of a nap. If you cannot sleep during the day because your situation doesn't allow it, be sure to get more sleep than usual for the next several nights.

HOW LONG TO NAP

Salvador Dali's method of jolting himself awake from napping may not be a refreshing respite for most people, but taking short, soothing naps of just ten to fifteen minutes can be extremely valuable. The ultimate luxury is to nap for as long as your body requires, waking naturally when you no longer need to sleep. Regular afternoon nappers often sleep from thirty to forty-five minutes, with a few extra minutes at each end to ease in and out of the restful state.

If you need more than an hour of sleep at midday, it is likely that you are simply not getting enough sleep and rest during the night to allow for full recovery. The sleep-deprived person could easily sleep the afternoon away. While there is benefit in attempting to catch up on missed sleep by napping, it is important to monitor how much sleep is needed during your naps as a method of evaluating if you are getting enough sleep each night.

REST

Allowing for adequate rest is a huge part of injury prevention, recovery, and overall health.

When you get adequate amounts of the four types of rest listed below, (which includes sleeping enough), your body is better able to maintain homeostasis.

The degree to which recovery from exertion can by achieved simply by resting is truly amazing. Almost all of the body's processes normalize when we relax in a restful state. Blood pressure, pulse rate, respiration rate, and temperature (among many other processes), all tend to drop to healthy lows while we rest. Regular resting supports the body in maintaining the equilibrium of homeostasis, the energy-conserving condition of the body.

Rest is relative: running is more restful than sprinting, and standing is more restful than walking. When engaged in intense activity—even just focused mental concentration—any break will provide a rest. Take advantage of the various types of breaks that are available to you so that you can maximize your participation in sufficient rest each day.

FOUR TYPES OF REST

The four main types of rest—physical, sensory, emotional, and physiological—are each equally important for health. To optimize recovery and heighten awareness so that injuries can be avoided, it is imperative to rest as much as is needed in each of these areas.

Physical Rest

Physical rest is usually what most of us think of first when we consider resting. We slow or stop physical activity in order to give our bodies a rest. Putting the muscles at rest, including the heart muscle, is the biggest factor of physical rest. During sleep we put the muscles into their deepest rest, but any time we relax horizontally we are in a fairly deep state of physical rest.

Sensory Rest

Comfort is key when it comes to resting our senses. Pleasant environmental conditions in terms of smells, sights, sounds, weather, tastes, and so on, provide us with sensory rest. A natural environment, or even scenes and sounds of them, are more restful to the senses than those of civilization. Rural environments promote a state of tranquility and restfulness that cannot be achieved in the city. A steady diet of bright lights, loud noises, fumes, or other environmental irritations reduces your ability to participate in sensory rest.

Emotional Rest

Inner confidence, poise, a calm attitude, self-esteem, and a cooperative attitude within yourself and from the people with whom you come into contact all contribute to your ability to achieve emotional rest. Fear, anxiety, doubt, worry, pain, grief, aggravation, and other emotional upsets reduce your state of emotional rest. When attempting to optimize recovery, from sports performance or from an injury, maximizing emotional rest is an important factor.

If you are distracted mentally or emotionally, you are less likely to successfully focus your full attention on your physical activities. This greatly increases your chances of sustaining an injury. Take time each day to practice developing emotional rest, and eventually this valuable state of being will be yours for a great majority of every day.

"Fear, anxiety, doubt, worry, pain, grief, aggravation, and other emotional upsets reduce your state of emotional rest."

Physiological Rest

There is only so much that can be done in terms of physiological rest. The glands, organs, and other structures of the body that are not directly involved in physical activity all demand fuel in order to function. There is little that can be done to affect the fuel needs of these structures, except for the organs of digestion.

As discussed earlier, digestion demands can range from relatively light to quite significant, depending upon the combination, quality, and quantity of foods eaten. Foods that digest easily, such as ripe fruit, provide a very light digestive demand. However, when we overeat, choose foods that are not within our biological range, or consume difficult-to-digest food combinations (such as complex-carbohydrate foods with animal-based foods), we significantly increase the body's physiological workload.

One method of quantifying your level of physiological rest is to check your pulse before and after a meal. Pulse rate is a good indicator of how much work your body is performing at any given time. Meals that take a long time to digest represent a greater physiological demand than meals that digest easily and rapidly. The more fuel one puts into the digestive processes, the less energy is available for the body to perform its healing and recovery role. Pulse rate can rise by ten to twenty beats per minute following a difficult-to-digest meal.

REST IS NOT ENOUGH

Many people mistakenly think that by resting more they can sleep less. This is not the case. The need for sleep remains a reality regardless of how much or how deeply we rest. People have, at times, remained awake for as long as a week, and sometimes even longer, but eventually everyone falls asleep.

Some people emphatically say "I'll sleep when I'm dead!" We can assume they believe that by minimizing sleeping they are maximizing living, yet nothing could be further from the truth. Cheating yourself of sleep and rest will eventually leave you in short supply of the vitality and health that makes life worth living. To enjoy life's adventures fully, begin by taking care of yourself—including getting enough rest and sleep. You will likely lengthen your life as well as create abundant health and energy with which to savor it.

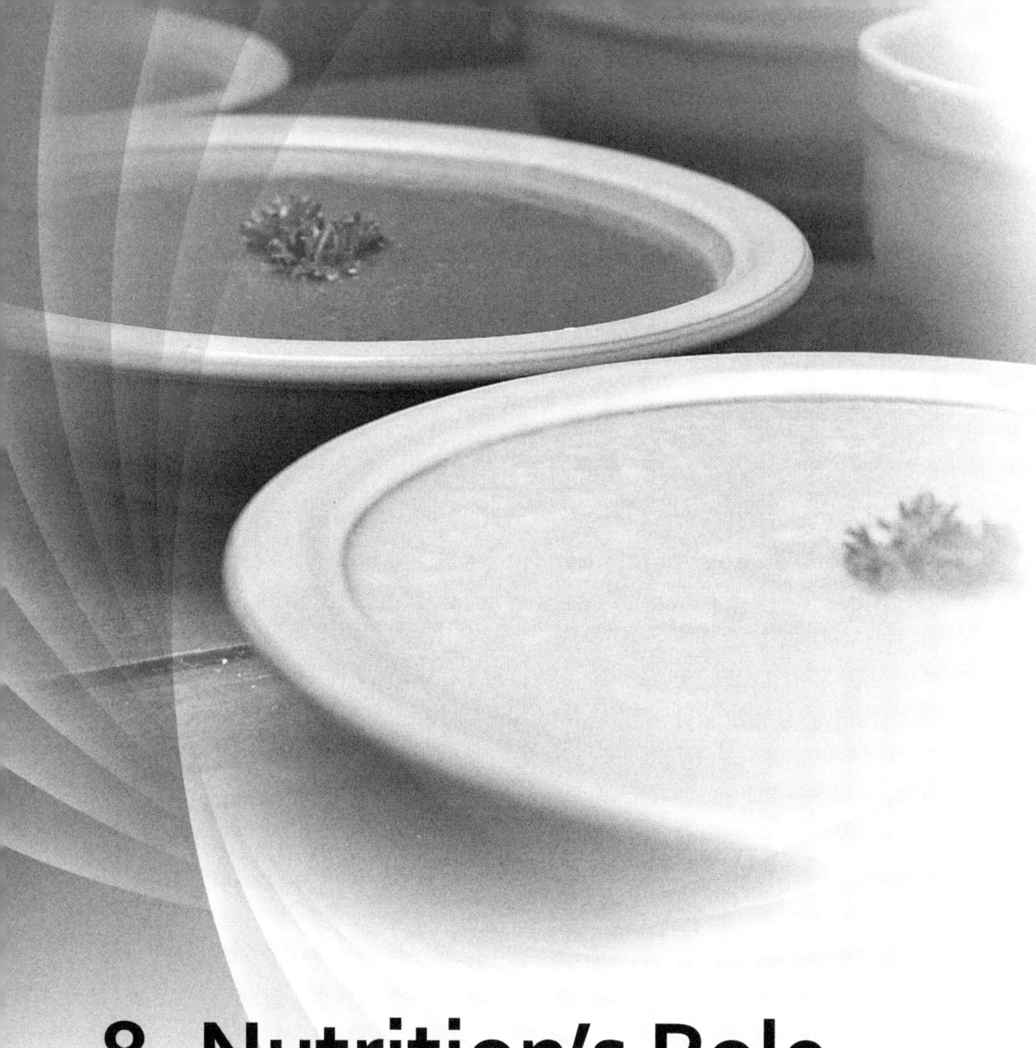

8. Nutrition's Role

When it comes to the prevention and care of injuries, it's easy to lose focus on the importance of nutrition. But its direct, immediate influence should not be underestimated. The role of nutrition is as important as any other in your training program. Well-nourished people heal more rapidly and tend to generate higher-quality tissue and bone than those who are undernourished.

If the weakest link in your prevention and recovery program happens to be nutrition, making small improvements in this area will help tremendously. And there are innumerable rewards for improving your nutrition beyond athletic recovery.

YOUR FUEL SUPPLY

No one would drive a car without checking the fuel gauge now and then. Learning to monitor and control your fuel supply is an essential aspect of every health program. When fuel levels go through dramatic ups and downs, you can experience symptoms that make you prone to injury. Sustained high blood-sugar levels inhibit healing and recovery of every type.

SIMPLE CARBOHYDRATES ARE THE PREFERRED FUEL

Carbohydrates are split into two categories: simple and complex. The complex sugars in plants are known as starches. Humans have several starch-splitting enzymes, the most well-known of which is ptyalin, the salivary amylase produced in the mouth. We do not produce much ptyalin, however, certainly not enough to digest raw complex carbohydrates, such as grains or tubers. Many foods containing starches include the carbohydrate group known as oligosaccharides, for which humans have no digestive enzymes at all. This makes the digestion of most complex carbohydrate foods literally impossible.

Simple Carbohydrates Require No Digestion

All the cells of our body are fueled by the simple sugar known as glucose, which is abundantly supplied in fruit. Approximately 90 percent of the body's cells will also accept another simple sugar found in fruit, known as fructose. Neither glucose nor fructose requires any digestion. These simple carbohydrates can be absorbed directly into the bloodstream from the small intestine and are immediately ready for use by the body.

Requiring no digestion is a huge plus when it comes to fuel efficiency. Directing energy to your brain functioning and recovery, instead of unnecessarily to digesting, results in greatly enhanced prevention and care of injuries. Easing the digestive demand can often mean the difference between a full daily recovery and overtraining.

"All the cells of our body are fueled by the simple sugar known as glucose, which is abundantly supplied in fruit."

The body converts simple carbohydrates into glycogen, a complex carbohydrate, and fills its "tanks" in the liver and the muscles. When we consume simple carbohydrates, they can be utilized directly by the muscles as fuel, or converted to glycogen for future use. All other fuels—complex carbohydrates, proteins, and fats—must be converted via digestion to simple carbohydrates in order to be utilized. The nerve energy required to digest these nutrients, making them into usable fuel, reduces their efficiency greatly. Much of the fuel supplied by foods other than simple carbohydrates is then used in the process of digesting them.

Simple Carbohydrates Are the Quickest Route to Refueling

Here is an example that will hopefully make things even clearer. Let's say that you have a machine that functions every time you put a penny into it. The machine's job is to digest, absorb, assimilate, and eliminate your food, so you want to keep this machine running. You have two sources of money: a tree that produces pennies and a bush that produces dollar bills. (If only it were so easy.) Collecting dollar bills is faster, for sure, but they cannot be used in your machine, which only accepts pennies. You decide to collect dollar bills anyway, and take them to the bank to have them converted into pennies.

Of course, the bank charges a fee for this service, so you only get 75 pennies in return for each dollar bill. By the time you return from the bank you make a startling realization. The time and energy (and pennies) spent going to the bank, getting a parking spot, paying the meter, waiting in line at the bank, dealing with the teller, counting out the pennies, and returning to your food machine was such a drain that you now only have a few pennies left.

In the long run it would have been much more efficient to simply collect and use pennies. But by now you are used to the process, so the next time you need money, you collect dollar bills and repeat the entire procedure.

The simple carbohydrates found in fruit, and in lesser quantities in vegetables, provide the ideal fuel for your body, in a readily acceptable form. Whole, fresh, ripe, raw, and organic, they come complete with the full package of essential nutrients known to be necessary for human health. Consuming fruit is the most efficient, effective, and healthful method of fueling your body.

Glycemic Concerns

The glycemic index is perhaps one of the most misunderstood and hence misinterpreted of all scientific indices. Simply stated, the glycemic index lists the rate at which carbohydrates from different foods enter the bloodstream (in the quantity of 50 grams). This is viewed as a simple but relatively accurate assessment of different foods' impact upon blood sugar.

In reality, many factors affect how quickly sugar enters the bloodstream, including but not limited to: current blood-sugar level, emotional state, level of rest, hydration, and others unique to the individual. A certain food may elicit quick and extreme blood-sugar responses in one person while the same food has just a minor effect upon another person.

Fruit is often thought of negatively because of its reputation for being a high-glycemic index food. This is an unfair assessment, as can be easily noted by reviewing a glycemic index chart. Foods are divided into three groups, rated for their low, moderate, and high glycemic response. Almost all of the high glycemic response foods are cooked complex carbohydrates, while the moderate and low groups are predominated by fruits. In reality, just because a food is high in sugar does not mean it creates a high glycemic effect. Fruit is simply the best choice for maintaining homeostasis in blood sugar and many other aspects of performance and recovery.

Raw Building Materials

The raw materials necessary for building a house—bricks, tiles, lumber, and so on—are themselves finished products, but they can be assembled into increasingly complex structures. A brick is not a house, obviously, but it is complete unto itself. It's a finished product comprised of many ingredients, and one that required construction itself. A house is also a finished product, even though it is likely to undergo a lifetime of additions, repairs, and remodeling. Our foods have a similar relationship to our bodies as do building materials to a house. Raw fruits and vegetables are finished products. They are constructed of many parts, known as nutrients.

When we eat them, our bodies deconstruct them to their smallest parts through the catabolic process known as digestion. Then the body utilizes the nutrients, as is, or reconstructs them as needed into increasingly complex structures. Growth and repair are the outcome of this reconstruction process.

Whole, ripe, raw foods are not "unfinished." They are complete and ready to be utilized. They require no preparation; no recipes are necessary for their consumption.

"Like all creatures on planet earth, our ancestors lived exclusively on a diet of raw foods through hundreds of millions of years of our evolutionary history. They grew ever-more intelligent and thrived on such fare, showing none of the signs of ill health that plague modern humans.

Slowly but surely, groups of humans scattered around the globe adopted cooking over the course of tens of thousands of years to allow them to survive in fruit-poor regions, or at times when proper raw food was unavailable in sufficient quantity. This change in diet has had little to no effect on our digestive anatomy. As a species, our nutritional requirements do not allow us to adapt to the consumption of cooked foods at all.

The influence of damaged, deranged and destroyed nutrients caused by cooking, the intake of mutagens and carcinogens created during the cooking process, and the lack of consumption of critical nutrients that is the inevitable result of changing from our natural diet to less-than-ideal foods rendered edible through the application of heat, can each only result in health decline and the eventual devolution of our species.

The quality of the home we build is directly related to the effectiveness of the building materials we choose. The healthiest foods for humans are those with nutrients that most closely match our nutritional needs: fruits, and secondarily, vegetables. More than any other food groups, whole, fresh, ripe, raw, organic fruits and vegetables provide us with all of the nutrients we require in order to develop optimum health.

Empty Calories and Junk Foods

Simple carbohydrates taste sweet, and are known as sugars. They come in two basic packages: whole and refined. Refined sugars, which are taken exclusively from plants, have been stripped of some or all of their accompanying nutrients and are accordingly referred to as "empty calories."

In truth, any calories that have been wholly or partially extracted from their rich nutrient package qualify to be properly identified as empty, and also as refined. The refining process is simply the removal of any nutrient from what was originally a whole food.

Remove the fiber from a grain and refined flour remains. Remove the fiber from a fruit or vegetable and a refined product known as juice remains. Remove the fiber (and also the water, carbohydrates, proteins, enzymes, co-enzymes, minerals, vitamins, phytonutrients and most of the anti-oxidants) from an olive, nut, seed, or vegetable and what is left is the highly refined, empty-calorie product known as oil.

"Junk food" refers to highly processed and chemical-laden foods, but also to foods that are comprised of mostly refined, empty calories. Because nutrients are destroyed in the cooking process, the calories that are left in all cooked foods have to be considered at least partially "emptied."

And because water is lost in the cooking process, cooked foods have to be considered refined, as well. Thus, even cooked foods that are usually considered nutritious begin to look a lot more like junk food once we realize that they are nothing more than refined, empty calories.

Top performance at any level of fitness requires the real thing when it comes to nutrition. Fruits have always been recognized as health foods. They are the source of nutrients that all manufacturers rely upon when they make their "healthy" products. Manufacturers of junk foods put catchphrases such as "with fruit sugar," "made with real fruit," "contains fruit," or "contains pectin and guar from fruit" on their labels in an attempt to link their products to the wholesomeness that is associated with fresh, whole fruit.

"A plant in need is early to seed," say the farmers, meaning that if a plant is stressed for what it requires (such as water), it will flower early in an effort to reproduce itself at all costs. We can see this axiom demonstrated in the early age at which our youngsters are now reaching puberty.

One hundred years ago, it was not uncommon for a woman to reach puberty around eighteen to twenty years of age. Today it is common for a girl to reach puberty before the age of twelve. The exaggerated height of today's teens, said to be a result of the growth hormones and antibiotics given to the animals whose meat and byproducts weigh heavily in many children's diets, is not matched by the additional calcium such height demands in order to create strong bones.

Rather, it is likely that the youth of today will become osteoporotic *before* their mothers. Many health experts are predicting that today's young people will develop cancer, heart disease, and diabetes earlier than previous generations did.

We cannot grow healthier than the quality of the foods we consume. The quality of cellular turnover—or the replacement of existing cells with new ones—is determined in great part by the quality and appropriateness of the foods we consume. If you wish to become healthier, you cannot choose better fuel than whole, fresh, ripe, raw, organic fruits and vegetables. Junk food cannot build a body that will remain healthy for a lifetime.

WATER CONSIDERATIONS

Proper hydration is a huge factor when it comes to fitness performance, recovery, and the healing of injuries. Most people are almost constantly dehydrated, at least to a mild degree. Insufficient water in your system impairs the thinking process, impedes coordination,

> **"We cannot grow healthier than the quality of the foods we consume."**

and slows recovery by negatively affecting your cells' ability to uptake nutrients and eliminate the toxic waste products of cellular metabolism. All body chemistry is adversely affected by dehydration.

As discussed in Chapter 6, there are three basic factors to consider when evaluating your level of hydration: frequency of urination, color of the urine, and the volume of urine expelled. It's essential that optimum levels of hydration be maintained as much as possible.

There are many types of water available on today's market, some more appropriate for human consumption than others. It is not within the scope of this book to discuss every type of water currently being marketed. To understand the complexity of the water issue, it may suffice to mention that water is the best-selling beverage in the United States.

The purpose of drinking is to rehydrate oneself. Pure water is best at fulfilling this function. Distilled water, condensed water, and reverse osmosis water are the best, in terms of quality. They add water and essentially nothing else to your system. Spring water is usually superior to mineral water, which is almost always better than tap water. Chlorinated, fluoridated, or otherwise chemically treated water, especially tap water, is generally the lowest quality potable water available.

Under healthful living conditions, humans actually do not have a high need for the consumption of free water. Due to varying weather, climactic, environmental, lifestyle, and fitness conditions, it is impossible to say, on average, how much water a human needs to consume. Certainly enough is required to stay well-hydrated.

When the weather complies, and lifestyle and diet supports it, a healthy human can easily go weeks and sometimes months without drinking any fluids while remaining well-hydrated. On the other hand, in extreme conditions, it is not unthinkable that an athlete might require a gallon of water per day.

"In extreme conditions, it is not unthinkable that an athlete might require a gallon of water per day."

Our anthropoid cousins—bonobos, gorillas, chimpanzees, orangutans, and others—rarely, if ever, drink water. They tend to be far fitter than we are in every way, too. Of course, staying well-hydrated is not only affected by how much water you consume. A diet high in fruits and vegetables, which are water-rich foods, has a profoundly positive influence upon hydration. But the biggest factor may be the avoidance of foods that result in thirst.

There are two classes of foods that will result in dehydration: foods that are toxic and foods that have had their water removed. Almost all condiments contain toxic ingredients. Cooking drives the water off of foods, making them dehydrated in almost all cases. The rare exceptions are the few foods that take on water when they are boiled, such as grain products that have been dehydrated prior to being cooked, such as pasta and oatmeal.

The consumption of cooked foods will therefore almost always result in excessive thirst. Dehydrated fruits, nuts, crackers, and other dried foods will also require copious quantities of water to be properly utilized. Any food that overtly results in thirst is worthy of question when it comes to optimum prevention and care of athletic injuries.

Dehydration essentially means "not enough water." Toxic chemicals in the body increase the need for water, for when it comes to body chemistry, "the solution to pollution is dilution." Excitotoxins, salt, food additives, and many artificial flavors and colors must be heavily diluted in order to be tolerated, increasing yet again our need for water consumption.

Whether from not enough water or too many toxins, dehydration can be effectively and safely handled by staying well-hydrated, regardless of the toxic load. Minimize the toxic load by reducing toxin intake and supplying the body with sufficient recovery time and conditions so that it detoxifies at the maximum degree possible.

Cooking also creates many toxic substances from the nutrients that are inherent within our foods. These toxins must be diluted if they are to be tolerated at all, thus increasing our need for water. The fact that almost everyone eats cooked food does not change the following facts: all cooking destroys nutrients and creates toxins.

THE INFLUENCE OF HEATED NUTRIENTS ON STRUCTURAL INTEGRITY

Almost every known nutrient is affected adversely by exposure to heat and is either damaged, deranged, or totally destroyed. The greater the heat and the longer the exposure, the worse the damage. Many nutrients, including fats and carbohydrates, actually become carcinogenic when exposed to heat, meaning that they become known cancer-causing agents. Others, including many antioxidants, phytonutrients, enzymes, co-enzymes, vitamins, and even some minerals, lose their anti-cancer qualities when heated, thus contributing to cancer's likelihood.

The enzyme-resistant bonds that form when proteins are heated make it impossible for the body to utilize their constituent amino acids in growth and repair processes. When fats are heated, their open, or unsaturated, bonds are often converted to triple, or closed, saturated bonds. This renders them unusable, as the body can only utilize fats that contain open, unsaturated bond sites. Enzymes and co-enzymes are deactivated at temperatures over 118°F, as are almost all nutrients that have a protein as part of their structure. Most vitamins lose their capacity to function once they have been subjected to a heat that surpasses 131°F.

While many nutrients in foods become inert due to exposure to the heat of cooking, most become toxic in some fashion. They become work for the body to process and eliminate—an excessive detoxification load for anyone desiring a speedy recovery from injury or even a normal recovery from the day's activities. Growth and development is inhibited due to the inaccessibility of various nutrients and the growth that does occur is often abnormal, showing signs of stress.

"While many nutrients in foods become inert due to exposure to the heat of cooking, most become toxic in some fashion."

HEATED COMPLEX CARBOHYDRATES

Heated carbohydrates are caramelized, with carcinogenic results. The more a carbohydrate is heated, the greater the negative outcome. When bread is toasted, for example, the change in its color represents the degree to which caramelization has taken place. Totally blackened bread is far more carcinogenic than bread that has been lightly toasted, but all exposure to carcinogens is toxic and contraindicated for health. Toxins such as these are kept in a dilute solution of water by the body to minimize the harm they do.

The nutritional value of complex carbohydrates is adversely affected by exposure to heat. Consumption of heated complex carbohydrates can influence human health in profoundly negative ways.

Adrenals: Phosphorus is leached from the adrenal glands as a response to the fermentation that often follows the consumption of complex carbohydrates, causing them to alternate between states of hyper- and hypo-activity. Headaches, foul body odor, lethargy and excessive mucus production are some symptoms of adrenal malfunction.

Thyroid: The by-products of fermentation—alcohol and acetic acid—are toxic to human cells. One of the responses of the body to acetic acid is hyperactivity of the thyroid. After a period of time the thyroid eventually "burns out" and goes hypo-active. Hypoactivity of the thyroid is a common problem in the Western world today.

Cellular Health: When complex carbohydrates are heated in the presence of fats, a toxin known as acrylamide is produced. Acrylamide is a known carcinogen, meaning that exposure to it or consumption of it results in cancer.

The increased consumption of complex carbohydrates has been touted as the solution to many of man's nutritional problems. While eating complex carbohydrates may be more nutritionally and environmentally sound than the consumption of animals, it falls far short of ideal when compared to eating the simple carbohydrates and other nutrients found in fresh fruit.

Mental acuity and all aspects of recovery are compromised when complex carbohydrates are consumed. Complex carbs often pose an extremely high digestive demand, have the highest glycemic index rating (as opposed to fruit, which rates in the middle or low range on the glycemic index), and most complex carbohydrates are known to contain chemical compounds known as opioids.

HEATED PROTEINS

The degree to which the skin inside your mouth can withstand hot water without damage gives you a rough idea of how much heat your food can withstand before the proteins begin to become damaged and denatured. Once denatured by exposure to heat, the damaged nutrients cannot ever be reconstructed into valuable ones. Like Humpty Dumpty, or an egg once it hits the frying pan, it "cannot be put together again."

The detrimental impact of heat on the proteins within your food cannot be overstated: enzyme-resistant bonds are formed, the proteins become denatured, toxins are created from what was once nutritious food, and the amount of available protein lessens the more the food is heated.

There is yet another feature of heated proteins that is worthy of our consideration when it comes to prevention and care of injuries, and that is the form they take when they actually enter the bloodstream. Ideally, proteins are broken down during the digestive process into smaller particles known as proteoles. Proteoles become polypeptides, and eventually these are digested into dipeptides. Dipeptides are very small, and can easily enter the digestive tract. At the liver, these dipeptides can be converted into individual amino acids and recombined as needed.

However, the enzyme-resistant bonds that form in heated proteins prevent our digestive enzymes from doing their job of breaking the polypeptides into smaller units. Some polypeptides enter directly into the bloodstream, while others enter via the lymphatic system. As they pass through the lacteals that serve as their portal of entry into the lymphatic system, the overly large particles damage these delicate tissues, enlarging the opening.

Over time, this repetitive damage prevents the lacteals from being as selective about which particles enter the lymphatic system. Similar damage occurs at the entry sites into the bloodstream. This inability to discriminate is known as "leaky gut syndrome." While leaky gut syndrome has many symptoms, primary among them are allergies, arthritis, digestive disorders, and various autoimmune conditions such as lupus.

Furthermore, when these partially digested proteins, known as polypeptides, enter the bloodstream, they are perceived as foreign invaders and are attacked by our white blood cells. The resulting "white tide," where the number of white blood cells multiplies by three to six times, is considered normal by most scientists. The proper name for this condition is *leukocytosis,* which refers to the increase of white blood cells in the blood. Extra water is held by the body to keep these toxins diluted.

HEATED FATS

Fats go through many changes when exposed to heat and none of them are positive, nutritionally. When fats are heated they become sticky. These sticky fats coat food particles making digestion less efficient. The sticky fat also coats the intestinal wall, impeding absorption of nutrients.

Once heated fats enter the bloodstream, they cause red blood cells to stick together in clumps. This reduces red blood cells' ability to uptake oxygen, which lowers our ability to participate in and recover from fitness activities. Heated fats in the bloodstream also increase the formation of a thrombi, a type of embolism that often results in heart attack or stroke.

"Once heated fats enter the bloodstream, they cause red blood cells to stick together in clumps. This reduces red blood cells' ability to uptake oxygen, which lowers our ability to participate in and recover from fitness activities."

In short, the chronic poor digestion caused by heated nutrients and junk foods leads to consistently poor rebuilding of cells, opening the door to injury and slowed healing and recovery.

NUTRITION AND INJURIES

As we discussed earlier, the quality of the building materials used in any construction project exerts a huge influence on the quality of the end product. This concept holds completely true for human growth, development, and repair. Low-quality tissues result when we consume empty calories, junk foods, and toxin-laden foods.

When subjected to the high-stress mechanics of sport and fitness activities, low-quality tissues are more prone to mechanical failure and injury than their high-quality counterparts.

People who are prone to repetitive injuries are often guilty of attempting to repair those injuries with nutrients from low-quality foods. Fresh, raw, organic fruits and vegetables supply the highest quality nutrients available. As we increase the percentage of these foods in our diet, the overall quality of our cells, tissues, organs, and systems will improve accordingly.

FUELING YOUR RECOVERY TO REDUCE INJURY SUSCEPTIBILITY

When we are physically active, certain key nutrients are utilized extensively and must be replaced. The sooner these nutrients are made available, the faster and better the recovery, and the lower the likelihood of injury. Of primary concern are the following nutrients: water, simple carbohydrates, and the minerals sodium and potassium.

Recovery is Hydrated

While water has already been discussed, it is also worth mentioning that adequate water must be available to the body in order to assimilate nutrients. It's a good idea to drink water before hard workouts if weather conditions are such that you will incur significant water losses.

If you are not sure how much water you lose during your typical workouts, you might try weighing yourself before and after a few training sessions, as previously mentioned. The weight loss incurred during a workout represents almost exclusively water weight. To replace the lost water, figure that each pint of water weighs approximately one pound, as mentioned in Chapter 6.

If you are feeling more tired than you would anticipate following a training session, consider the possibility that you may be dehydrated. It is better to err on the side of caution and drink an extra glass or two of water, than to slow recovery by experiencing the deleterious effects of dehydration.

Recovery is Sweet

Simple carbohydrates are often the missing nutritional link when it comes to optimum athletic recovery. The best source of simple carbohydrates is fresh fruit. We don't need much practice to train ourselves to eat sweet, fully ripened fruit after physical activity, especially because the results are so positive.

The simple sugars that predominate in fruit, glucose and fructose, are used to refuel the muscles after exercise. These simple, readily assimilated carbohydrates are quickly converted into muscle glycogen. Muscle function and recovery is greatly dependent upon this process.

Recovery is Salty

Sodium is the main extracellular mineral, potassium the main intracellular mineral. Functioning as electrolytes (minerals that carry an electrical charge), sodium and potassium are instrumental to the cell's ability to uptake nutrients and eliminate metabolic waste products. These two minerals must stay in proportion to each other in order for the cell to maintain structural and functional integrity. If there is too much sodium in the extracellular fluid, it will pull water out of the cells and dehydrate them, disrupting cellular function.

Although extremely uncommon, it's possible, to have too much potassium relative to sodium. This too would upset the cell's mineral balance. The most common scenario that creates this condition is when we sweat profusely during a bout of extended physical exertion, such as the running of a marathon. Sodium is lost with our perspiration. If not replaced, sodium levels can eventually go so low that potassium is pulled from the cells in an attempt to maintain cellular electrolytic balance.

As potassium leaves the cells, weakness, nausea, cramping, and eventually total prostration will ensue. Fortunately, such a condition is extremely uncommon as human physiology adapts in just a few days to high-sodium losses by conserving this important mineral.

The quantity of sodium and potassium found in fresh fruits and vegetables meets human nutritional needs quite closely. Cooked foods, dried foods, and most other bottled, boxed, frozen, canned, and bagged foods contain added salt. The salt functions as a preservative, extending the shelf life of the food while shortening ours.

If a shipwrecked man drinks seawater, he'll soon die. The dehydration caused by the salt (sodium chloride) in the water is more than a person can bear. To remove the salt from seawater and then eat it would seem the height of insanity. Yet this is exactly what most people typically do, consuming on average more than twenty times the amount of salt per day than they require.

An extended shelf life for food is definitely a negative quality when it comes to human nutrition. The longer the shelf life of a food, the less likely that it can be consumed by microbes. A great majority of our digestive processes depend upon the catabolic influence of microbes upon our food. Food that doesn't support microbes literally does not support life.

While we tend to think of foods being consumed by microbes as having "gone bad," the reality is that only foods that are good for us can actually "go bad." Foods that cannot go bad simply cannot provide vital human nutrition. Thus, length of shelf life generally indicates how inert a food is, and the more inert, the less nutritious.

Depending upon the source of the sodium, salt can also function as an excitotoxin. The sodium taken from soybeans in the manufacturing of various salty liquids, pastes, and bouillon for example, is rich in monosodium glutamate. Dr. Russell L. Blaylock, author of *Excitotoxins,* considers MSG to be the most damaging of all excitotoxins.

PROTEIN MYTHS ABOUT HEALING FROM INJURIES

In the wild, if an animal is injured or ill, it will often simply crawl under a bush or into a hole and safely wait for nature to take its course. Usually, within a few days, the body will heal itself. In the case of a severe wound or a broken bone, healing could take several weeks. No food is eaten during this time, as none is necessary, nor is it likely to be obtainable.

This method of healing is the most rapid and thorough that nature has devised. In order to direct energy to the processes of healing after injury, the body must redirect energy from somewhere else. Reducing physical (muscular) and physiological (digestive) activity frees a great deal of energy that the body can use to focus on its healing efforts.

When not feeling their best, animals usually stop eating. There is no way to persuade an animal to eat when it doesn't want to. Similarly, when humans do not feel well, we also lose our appetite. Nature provides us with many clues that food is not needed in order for us to heal from acute injuries and we would do best to abstain from eating.

There is protein in every cell of our bodies. Some of it is structurally integrated (stabile), and some is not (labile). Protein is utilized for all of the many repair functions carried out by the body, and that having sufficient protein available is essential. Fortunately, the body maintains more than half of its total protein in the form of labile proteins that are not structurally integrated. Since stabile proteins are not available for use during the body's repair procedures because they are structurally integrated, only the labile proteins are utilized.

Although little research has been done in this area, it shows clearly that recovery time from injury or sickness is shortened when food intake is reduced. While many medical doctors are currently teaching that more protein is better, especially in the case of healing, research and practical results do not support this opinion.

Wound and bone healing have been shown to progress at their most rapid rates when no food is consumed at all, as per the model demonstrated by animals in the wild. We know that muscular recovery after physical exertion is dependent upon a sufficiency of carbohydrate availability and not upon that of proteins. For long-term

"For long-term muscular growth, adequate protein is certainly a necessity, but there is virtually no evidence to date indicating that an excess of protein is more beneficial than the 5–10 percent of calories that have been shown to be adequate amounts."

muscular growth, adequate protein is certainly a necessity, but there is virtually no evidence to date indicating that an excess of protein is more beneficial than the 5–10 percent of calories that have been shown to be adequate amounts.

As for the concept that it is essential to have protein-rich foods in order to be healthy, several responses are appropriate. First, it must be realized that in order for any food to grow, it must contain protein. Protein is in the nucleus of every cell of everything alive. All whole foods, including fruits and vegetables, contain protein, as they are all made of cells.

We must consider that bulls, elephants, rhinoceroses, and other large, muscular vegetarian animals get their protein from the consumption of leafy greens. Anthropoids and other primates obtain a great deal of their protein from fruit. There is no reason to believe that a diet predominated by fruits and vegetables would somehow result in a protein deficiency in humans or that an excess of protein is in any way desirable.

NUTRITION AND TRAINING RESPONSE

To put it simply, protein, fat, and carbohydrates are the only three nutrients that supply us with the fuel that is otherwise known as calories. While any of these "caloronutrients" can be converted into the carbohydrate that the body uses for fuel, the simple carbohydrate sugars, glucose and fructose, are the preferred fuels of our cells.

It's relatively easy to figure out what percentage of calories need to come from protein, fat, and carbohydrates to best serve our nutritional and recovery needs. The math has been done for us, countless times, by many of the world's leading nutritionists, sports physiologists, and health experts.

Nutrition recommendations from the experts can often seem complicated, with different ratios of micro and macro nutrients handed out for different athletic pursuits. But in the run up to the 2000 summer Olympics in Sydney, when U.S. Olympic Committee Nutrition Coordinator Judy Nelson was asked to distill the often-complicated nutrition advice handed out to U.S.

Olympic athletes into a simple-to-understand formula, she explained that the easiest way to think of our needs was to remember the amount of calories required might vary widely from athlete to athlete, but the percent of their calories derived from fat, protein, and carbohydrates shouldn't change much.

"Most recreational athletes, and people interested in good health, will fall in the sixty percent carbohydrate, fifteen percent protein, twenty-five percent fat ballpark." Nelson said. "If you are lifting weight, you will need a little more protein, but that doesn't mean you'll need more protein than you're already eating. Most Americans easily get more protein than they need. If you're lifting weight and not getting muscle development, you may not be getting enough calories."

While protein has been touted as the quintessential nutrient, the imperative substance that must be consumed regularly and in great quantity, the overwhelming majority of health authorities and organizations agree that 10 percent of total calories from protein is more than sufficient. In fact, it is readily admitted that the suggestion of 10 percent allows for a substantial "margin of safety."

Certainly we don't see protein deficiency in the United States, where the average protein consumption is around 15 percent, nor among the elite Kenyan runners, who take in an average of 10.1 percent of their calories from protein. Protein's importance to our overall health has been greatly overstated, as has its availability.

With only two caloronutrients left to discuss, it becomes obvious that as the consumption of one goes up the other must go down. We have been urged for over four decades to increase our consumption of carbohydrates and decrease our consumption of fats. Now that the relationship of one to the other is clear, let's focus on how much fat we actually need.

A huge number of the world's nutritionists and health experts implore us to lower our total fat intake. Many suggest that our total fat intake should not exceed single digits as a percentage of total calories consumed, while most of the others say that our fat intake should hover in the teens.

If we take an average, it comes close to 10 percent. Most people are shocked to learn the average fat consumption per calorie in the United States is over 30 percent.

While we refer to flesh, fowl, dairy, and seafood as protein foods, along with nuts and seeds, almost all of these foods provide more than half—and many more than three-quarters—of their total calories in the form of fat. They should not be referred to as protein foods at all, as that designation must be saved for foods whose predominating caloronutrient is protein. Anything else is simply misleading.

With protein and fat consumption both averaging around 10 percent, it is easy to see that carbohydrate consumption is optimal when it ranges close to 80 percent of total calories consumed. We need to lower our fat consumption in order to raise our carbohydrate intake. The US national average for simple and complex carbohydrate consumption combined comes in at less than 50 percent of calories.

Insufficient carbohydrate consumption invariably leads to a profound lack of energy, as seen in people with Chronic Fatigue Syndrome/Myalgic Encephalopathy, and has been related to conditions ranging from candida overgrowth and diabetes to cancer, heart disease, and most digestive disorders. (For an in-depth understanding of these and many of the other caloronutrient concerns, see my book on this topic, *The 80/10/10 Diet.*)

Because of their bland flavor, complex carbohydrate foods generally require added salt (or other toxic condiments), refined sugar, or large quantities of fat. Thus, they cannot be the optimum

"Treat yourself to the best and eat fruit as a meal, all you care for, rather than just as a snack. Remember, fruit has always been considered a health food."

choice of fuel for human performance. (I have written extensively on this subject in my book, *Grain Damage.*)

Fruit, on the other hand, supplies the ideal source of fuel for all fitness needs. Fruits digest easily and quickly, release copious quantities of water, provide readily assimilated simple carbohydrates, are rich in all nutrients known to be important to human nutrition, and offer a healthy ratio of potassium to sodium.

Before a strength-training workout, during long-distance and endurance training, and after virtually all types of physical activity, fruit makes the ideal high-performance food. Treat yourself to the best and eat fruit as a meal, all you care for, rather than just as a snack. Remember, fruit has always been considered a health food.

RUNNING ON EMPTY

Active individuals need to maintain optimum blood-sugar levels if they want reliable performance results. The best results come when blood-sugar levels remain in a relatively tight range rather than going through huge swings. When your blood-sugar level drops, it is likely that your muscles are about to run out of their preferred fuel source: carbohydrates. While the body can create new sugar from fat when carbohydrate intake lags behind actual needs (via a process known as *gluconeogenesis*—literally, the creation of new sugar), it is an energy-intensive process and less efficient than directly fueling up on simple carbs from fruit.

Measuring blood sugar is the easiest method of evaluating fuel availability, and it's a relatively simple test to do. While not a perfect science, it is sufficiently accurate so that diabetics can use it as their standard method. It's not necessary for a healthy person to regularly monitor blood sugar via the use of a glucometer. Once one gets a feel for how blood sugar responds to different degrees of physical activity and the consumption of various foods by using a glucometer, personal blood-sugar levels become relatively easy to predict.

Results of Poor Fueling

Injuries related to low levels of fuel during physical activity mostly happen due to clumsiness. When people are running "on fumes," they are pushing themselves beyond their natural safety net. Marathon runners coined the phrase, "hitting the wall," to express just what it feels like to continue running once their blood-sugar levels start to drop and they are waiting for gluconeogenesis to provide new sugar from fat stores. To hit a wall and continue running through it is quite a feat. But there is no need to push oneself to such extremes in the pursuit of health and fitness. In fact, we are more likely to become healthy and fit from physical exertion when we maintain homeostasis than when we force huge metabolic swings.

Full Cells, Empty Tummy

While simple sugar enters the blood relatively easily and rapidly from the intestinal tract, it then moves into the muscles much more slowly. A functional level of sugar is maintained in the form of glycogen, a complex sugar, in the muscles. During extreme exertions, it's possible to have blood-sugar levels that are relatively high but muscles that are drained of most of their glycogen.

This is a scenario that usually will happen in less than two hours of all-out exertion. For a person with more experience in fitness training, it is likely that blood-sugar levels will run low as a result of more efficient fueling of the muscles. In this case, it is likely to take three to four hours of moderate exertion before fuel levels become exhausted.

Most people find that participating in intense endurance activities will result in nausea unless they start out with an empty or nearly empty stomach. Digestion and physical exertion simply do not work well together simultaneously. The ideal arrangement for exercise of almost any type has the blood sugar topped off, the cells fully loaded, and the stomach completely empty.

But to achieve such a state, muscles must be allowed to refuel from the prior day's activities. This can only be realized when sufficient simple carbohydrates are consumed—preferably from fruits. Any other food requires too much time and digestive effort to be efficient, or is missing vital nutrients. Favoring fruits is one of the healthiest steps we can take when it comes to proper fueling, nutrition, and recovery.

CARBOHYDRATE-LOADING: EXPLODING THE MYTH

Humans can store fat; in fact, we are very good at it. But we simply have no ability to store carbohydrates or protein, as physiologists and scientists have proven. If excess calories from protein are consumed, they are converted to fat for storage in the body. The same is true for carbohydrates. (In cases of compromised health, it's possible for protein and carbohydrates to be eliminated via the urine, as well.) We must therefore take a serious look at the concept that has been promoted as carbohydrate-loading.

A good analogy is the functional level of gasoline in the gas tank of a car. A car has no ability to store excess gasoline. It would be a disaster to pour it anywhere but into the tank. If you tried to put too much gas into the tank, it would spill over. In fact, "spill over" is the exact terminology used in the medical profession to describe what happens when we consume excess carbohydrates. They either "spill over" into the urine or they are converted to fat for storage.

We have a functional level of carbohydrates in our muscle cells, liver, and blood. Much like the amount of gasoline in your car's tank, this level can vary within an acceptable range. Too much and carbohydrates spill over; too little and we run out of fuel.

In the United States, people eat about 48 percent of their total calories from carbohydrates; a little more than half of what most health experts now recommend as ideal. An increase in dietary carbohydrates toward recommended levels will result in health and performance improvements. Carbohydrate-loading for a meal or two

"In the United States, people eat about 48 percent of their total calories from carbohydrates; a little more than half of what most health experts now recommend as ideal."

before a competition will therefore result in improved performance, simply by virtue of your coming closer to actually meeting your body's daily carbohydrate needs.

Perhaps the name just needs to be changed. If it were called "carbohydrate supplying" it would be more accurate and less misleading. If it were called, "giving the body what it has needed all along," the name would be right but no one would want to live with the truth that we don't usually give our bodies what they need.

The most nutritionally healthful method of eating is to supply adequate amounts and types of carbohydrates in the diet at all times. When that is the case, overall health and performance improve and carbohydrate-loading is not an issue. We can enter into fitness and physical activities with our liver, blood, and muscles fully supplied with all the carbohydrates necessary for top performance.

PROBLEMS WITH FAT CONSUMPTION

Fat has gotten a bad name, and not altogether undeservedly. Essential fatty acids (EFAs) are so named because they must be consumed in order for us to experience health. EFAs are found in all whole fruits and vegetables. Current research indicates that a plant-based diet that supplies 5–10 percent of its total calories as fat will provide us with the proper quantities of EFAs to match our needs. However, insufficient fat consumption is an extremely uncommon problem, while excess fat in the diet is epidemic.

A few of the relevant problems associated with too much fat in the diet include, but are not limited to, increases in: heart disease, cancer rates, diabetes rates, and chronic fatigue.

In fitness, the latter is our primary concern. Following is a brief overview of the mechanisms involved. Dietary fat moves through the digestive system more slowly than any other nutrient, whereas dietary sugars are only surpassed by water in their speed of passage and uptake. When fat is included with dietary sugars, the uptake of those sugars into the bloodstream is slowed. While the slower uptake of sugar means that we will experience delayed access to the fuel that it provides, it also means that the sugars are likely to ferment in our digestive tract. Fermentation of sugars in the digestive tract leads to a host of health problems, including: candida overgrowth, symptoms of drunkenness, cirrhosis (hardening of the liver), and thyroid dysfunction.

Excess dietary fat results in high quantities of fat in the bloodstream, where it wreaks havoc on sugar metabolism. The fat coats the sugar molecules as well as the insulin that attaches to them, making it difficult for the two to "hook up." This results in a condition known as "insulin-resistant diabetes," which generally resolves when fat intake is lowered to healthful levels. Because high levels of fat in the bloodstream hinder the muscles' ability to uptake sugars, they slow recovery from exercise and leave the consumer feeling sluggish. (For a more in-depth discussion of this and related topics, see my book, *The 80/10/10 Diet.*) Chronic fatigue results when the adrenal glands also become exhausted as a result of the above scenario. Fatigue either leaves you too tired to exercise or prone to injury if you do.

After any physical exertion, the best food is fresh fruit. Fats may be satiating, and may be what you are used to, but if you are looking for the best in terms of nutrition, fruit is definitely the food of choice after exercise. Fatty foods should be eaten in small quantities only, so that the fats comprise an average of about 10 percent of total calories consumed. As fats digest slowly, it is best not to eat them if you expect to be active shortly following their consumption. For these reasons, I recommend that fat consumption be reserved for the last meal of the day only.

Fuel on the Run

Sports drinks, electrolyte replacement fluids, energy drinks, and many other specialty substances are being increasingly marketed to a public that seems ever more eager to consume them. Somehow we have come to believe that there is a need for these products, even while we know that our grandparents did quite well without them, and that they exerted themselves physically to a much greater degree than we ever will. What is the solution to this apparent contradiction?

The answer lies in whether you choose to treat the symptoms

or to eliminate their cause. On a low-carbohydrate diet, the addition of carbohydrate-rich food will greatly enhance overall physical performance. (The average person in the United States consumes less than two thirds of the calories from carbohydrates that s/he requires—48 percent of total calories consumed as compared to the 80 percent that is recommended.)

On a diet that is exceedingly high in salt, additional water will enhance overall physical performance. (The average person in the United States consumes close to a month's worth of salt on a daily basis.)

On a diet of refined foods and a gross inadequacy of fresh vegetables, electrolyte replacement will enhance overall physical performance. (Almost all of the food in the standard Western diet has been refined in some way with the exception of whole fresh raw fruits and vegetables.) Eating a low-fat diet that is predominated by raw fruits and vegetables will largely eliminate the need for such products.

Water, carbohydrates, potassium, and sodium are the key needs when it comes to exercise-related nutrients. Water is often in the lowest relative supply of the four, and usually needs to be replenished before the others become an issue.

For relatively short stints of activity, forty-five minutes to an hour or less, no special considerations are generally necessary, other than being sure to be well-hydrated when you begin, and to finish the activity with a carbohydrate-rich meal, preferably of fresh fruit. Fruit will supply the carbohydrates, water, and potassium that are typically lost from within the cells during exercise.

For activities that are likely to range from an hour to ninety minutes, it is a good idea to bring water with you, or at least to know where it will be available. Water is the primary concern for exertions of this duration. Again, following up with a meal of fresh fruit is ideal.

If you are planning to exercise for more than ninety minutes, especially if the intensity level is going to be relatively high, fuel availability can become a consideration as well as water. It is a good idea to take along a couple of dates, or water that has had dried fruit soaked in it overnight.

For longer events of two hours or more, electrolytes can become an issue. Primarily of concern are the minerals potassium and sodium. Water, carbohydrates, and potassium must be replenished in the cells. Fruit is the best source for all three of these essential nutrients. If weather conditions favor heavy perspiration, there can be particularly heavy losses of sodium. In that case, include the consumption of green vegetables, especially celery, which is one of the richest sources of sodium of all vegetables.

Celery blends into fruit shakes very nicely, and is a surprisingly welcome addition to any meal. One bite of banana and one bite of celery provide more of the essential sports-related nutrients (except for water) than an entire bottle of even the most expensive commercial sports drinks could provide.

Should your exertions be longer than just a few hours—for example, if you have to do a large construction job or plan to take a multi-day bicycle trip—it is important to make sure that water, fresh fruit, and celery are readily available. These staples will supply your fuel and nutrient needs for all activities and will provide the ideal nutrient mix for speedy recovery.

REFUELING YOUR MUSCLES

The basic fuel of every cell is glucose, a simple carbohydrate. Getting this nutrient to your muscle's cells is the main goal of refueling. Finding the simplest and most energy-efficient method of doing so encourages efficient and effective recovery. A huge part of recovery involves refueling the muscles after their glycogen supplies have been used up during physical exertions.

When considering recovery, it is important to take into account the muscular growth that occurs as a response to strength training. Providing ideal conditions for refueling and growth are therefore the main goals for optimizing recovery.

Refueling with junk food, empty calories, or refined foods simply does not make sense, as they do not contain the essential nutrients required to healthfully assimilate the calories that we consume. The damage done to those calories by the cooking process only exacerbates the problem. Consuming cooked food seems even less appealing if you wish to recover healthfully and rapidly. It's much like building a house of out low-quality materials: the house can be built, but it will not stand up to much stress.

NUTRITION AND THE CYCLE OF ATHLETIC PROGRESSION

Athletes are always looking for an edge. Newer and higher standards in nutrition, coaching-training, and equipment, all play a role in improving performance, and through the years many new athletic records have been set due to the impact of these improvements.

Notice the role that nutrition has played in encouraging advancement in the other areas (see the discussion below). Progress in each area has certainly dovetailed with the others, but for the most part, nutrition led the pack.

During the twentieth century, in the '60s and into the '70s, changes in nutritional emphasis played a major role in enhancing athletic performances. Though "meat and potatoes" had long been considered the best athletic fare, the meat was often favored over the potatoes. The tide was turning, however, and complex carbohydrates were gaining favor among forward-thinking athletes.

Several athletes from different parts of the world found that their performance improved noticeably when they consumed more complex carbohydrates instead of fatty or high-protein foods. Those who refused to keep up with the times nutritionally were left in the dust on the playing field.

In the '80s, athletes running on these more efficient fuels started to demand better equipment. Technology responded with a wave of plastic, fiberglass, polycarbonate, aluminum, titanium, and graphite equipment that was stronger, lighter, and better attuned to accommodate and even encourage improved performance.

Safety concerns were also being addressed and training became safer through inflatable landing pits, overhead safety harnesses, more efficient padding (i.e. pads for in-line skating and related sports were introduced), and a wide assortment of coach/athlete communication devices.

The '90s brought huge changes in coaching strategies. Athletes were better nourished and using more sophisticated equipment, and coaches found that they could push them to new performance heights.

By employing advanced training strategies—plyometrics, unstable training surfaces, resistance bands, and drag training—for their athletes, coaches pushed competitors to their max. A huge array of technological advances also made teaching more efficient, monitoring performance more objective, and training more effective.

With the dawning of the new millennium came a renewed urgency on the part of athletes to gain an edge over their competition. Diet became the focus once more, as equipment and coaching advantages were few and far between. Industry continued to market to athletes, and nonathletes alike, a vast array of drinks, goos, gels, butters, powders, and bars that would supposedly enhance athletic performance, but "better living through chemistry" didn't hold true when it came to enhanced athletic performance, especially not in the long run.

Fruit is catching on in the world of sports. Top performers gravitate to the best lifestyle choices for health and fitness, and fruit is the absolute best when it comes to sports nutrition. No amount of flashy marketing or hype can hide the fact that fruit provides athletes the simplest, cleanest, and most efficient form of fuel possible, while being the tastiest and most enjoyable. This century, sports records are being broken and will continue to be as athletes realize that the healthier they eat, the better they feel, heal, and perform.

NUTRITION AND RECOVERY

OVERTRAINING

When it comes to refueling and recovering, overtraining can pose a serious and major encumbrance. The body can only create a limited amount of glycogen in any twenty-four hour period. When overtraining, especially for many hours, it becomes impossible for the muscles to take on enough sugar for the next day's activities. When muscles are underrecovered in terms of sugar uptake, performance becomes sluggish and there is increased risk of injury.

WEIGH, WEIGH, WEIGH

Fat loss through physical training is usually slow unless you are exceptionally fit. You need to run thirty-five miles to burn the calories in just one pound of fat. Most people are simply not fit enough to rapidly lose excess fat solely through exercise. A combination of diet and exercise will invariably work best.

Water-weight loss, on the other hand, can be extremely rapid during a workout. As mentioned earlier, one pint of water weighs one pound. It is not unusual to lose four to six pounds or more of water weight during a workout where you perspire freely. Unless this water is replaced quickly after the exercise session is finished, recovery will be greatly hampered, as the necessary nutrients cannot be carried into the cells without sufficient water being available.

In order to ensure that you are well-hydrated, see the guidelines listed in Chapter 6 under the heading, "Hydration."

PROTEIN AND RECOVERY

Somehow, protein seems to be ranked highest on the list of important nutrients. People tell me that they eat meat or cheese because they "crave protein." (Of course, the predominating nutrient in meat and cheese is fat, not protein.) Our perception of well-rounded nutrition is skewed to favor protein, as if protein can do no wrong. This simply is not the case. Sufficient protein is necessary, but an excess of it is a problem, as it is with any nutrient. As mentioned earlier, according to most experts, sufficient protein translates to about 5–10 percent of total calories consumed. Once again, more is not better.

"Sufficient protein translates to about 5–10 percent of total calories consumed. Once again, more is not better."

Protein's importance to our overall health has been greatly overstated, as has its availability. In most situations, about 0.25 percent of the total fuel used in fitness pursuits comes from protein. If a person walks four miles, he or she would have used less than one calorie in protein for fuel. This 0.25 gram of protein can easily be regained by eating just a bite or two of a banana. The idea that protein is used for recovery is not completely false, though. Protein's primary role in the body is for growth and repair.

If there is damage done to the body during a workout, protein is needed to help in the repair process. If muscles are challenged for strength, growth will be the outcome, and again, protein will be used. Taking this into account plus allowing for the fact that not all protein consumed is necessarily absorbed, and then raising the total requirement slightly more at the end just to be sure, we still find that less than 10 percent of total calories from protein is sufficient. Since fruits average about seven percent protein and vegetables average about 20 percent protein, it becomes obvious that a diet of fresh fruits and vegetables makes protein deficiency an impossibility.

Recovery is optimized when our nutritional needs are most closely met. By supplying 80 percent of total calories from carbohydrates, we limit the amount of protein available in the diet to about 10 percent. Once this is understood, we can let go of the false idea that the body heals and recovers best when high-protein foods are consumed. Infants show the fastest growth rate of all humans, and they do so while consuming nothing but mother's milk, a food whose protein content is listed as only six percent of total calories.

If we take care of our predominant nutrient needs for recovery by eating fruit—water, simple carbohydrates, and potassium—we will also meet our protein needs.

Putting Protein Concerns to Rest

"But where do you get your protein?" Vegetarians typically explain that they get sufficient protein from the whole foods they consume, as anything that grows must have protein in it. (Protein is, in fact, integrated into the structure of every living cell.) Vegans explain that they get their protein from the plant foods they consume, just like vegan animals do.

And raw foodists explain that there is plenty of protein in fruits and vegetables. With everyone explaining the protein issue so often, it is amazing that it is even still is an issue. Protein concerns are deeply ingrained. Despite all of the explaining, and despite all evidence to the contrary, many people still end up thinking, "Yeah, but I am still not sure about getting enough protein." The funny thing is that people on the standard American diet only manage to take in 15 percent of their calories from protein, despite all the supposedly protein-rich animal foods they're consuming.

The Function of Protein

Protein is primarily used for growth and repair. Growth and repair each play a part in recovery from injury and from daily workouts. In reality, however, the body does not use protein, per se, but uses amino acids, the "building blocks" of protein. There are 20 different amino acids that are used in the human body to make proteins.

There can be anywhere from 50 to 27,000 amino acids in a protein, although most proteins are around a few hundred amino acids in length. To be properly digested, proteins must be broken down several times until eventually individual amino acids result. These amino acids are then recombined to form the protein structures needed by the body.

The body maintains a "pool" of amino acids, kept ready and waiting to be utilized as needed. We don't need any specific amino acid to be consumed at any given meal or on a specific day, as the pool is large enough to allow for such variance. Fortunately, you do not have to keep track of all of this growth and repair as your body takes care of it for you, perfectly. All you have to do is eat, exercise, and sleep.

"Fortunately, you do not have to keep track of growth and repair as your body takes care of it for you, perfectly. All you have to do is eat, exercise, and sleep."

Sources of Protein

Protein is found in the DNA of all living cells. DNA is found in the nucleus of every cell, and is considered to be the "brain" or "blueprint" from which the cell functions. Unless the protein has been refined out of it, any food that was once alive is a source of protein. Of course, cooking the food makes the protein less available.

The fact is, we need less protein than we tend to think we do. The average protein intake in the United States is around 15 percent of total calories consumed. If we say that the average man consumes about 3,000 calories and the average woman about 2,000 calories per day, that would mean their protein consumption was 450 calories (112 grams) and 300 calories (75 grams) respectively.

As mentioned, some percentage of that protein became nonviable when it was cooked, but some remained bioavailable. Just how much of the protein becomes nonviable is anyone's guess, and is dependent to a great degree on the amount of heat used in the cooking. And as stated earlier, we do know, however, that 6 percent of calories from protein supplies enough of this vital nutrient to meet all of a growing baby's protein needs, as that is the amount in mother's milk.

Fruits' protein content ranges from about 4–10 percent of total calories. Vegetables have a larger range, about 10–50 percent of calories, but typically contain about 20 percent protein. Nuts and seeds also yield almost 20 percent of their calories from protein. If 10 percent of the day's calories came from vegetables, 10 percent from nuts and seeds, and the other 80 percent from fruit, the protein content for a typical day would be very close to 10 percent.

Even on a diet of just fruit (not recommended) we would likely average about 7 percent protein, more than is found in mother's milk. When eating whole foods, it is actually difficult to underconsume protein.

Where we run into trouble is when we consume empty calories such as refined sugar, refined flour, alcohol, or oil. These calories provide no protein whatsoever. Meals made from these refined substances tend to be correspondingly low in protein. Even so, it is exceptionally rare to find protein deficiency even in a person who eats sweets and breads, uses oils, and drinks alcohol.

Once again, whole, fresh, ripe, raw organic fruits and vegetables provide us with all the nutrients we need, in exactly the proportions in which we need them. Let these foods predominate your diet and hopefully you will now feel comfortable putting the entire protein issue to rest.

Too Much or Not Enough?

Many supporters of high-protein diets do not realize how harmful excessive proteins are to the body. They suggest that we need to eat lots of protein toward the end of the day or else the body will begin devouring itself before morning. This is unfounded, for as we have determined, the body uses primarily carbohydrates, not protein, for fuel, and fuel use during the night is relatively low.

Some body builders say they have a special need for protein for fuel. They are correct if, and only if, they do not supply themselves with sufficient carbohydrates to use for fuel. In that instance, the body will utilize protein as a fuel source, but it is extremely inefficient at doing so. It would be far easier on the body to supply the necessary carbohydrates, rather than consume proteins, and then have the body work to convert them into carbohydrates.

The low-carbohydrate diets that are currently extremely popular are also extremely dangerous. Any time we remove a major calorie source from our diet, we are likely to lose weight, so in that sense these diets do work. But the price is great. Liver failure, kidney failure, and heart failure are all common on low-carbohydrate diets. Too much protein is a much more likely problem than not enough.

It is wise to learn how to supply your nutritional needs to best support your fitness performance and overall recovery. (For further coverage of this topic, refer to my book, *Nutrition and Athletic Performance*).

NUTRIENTS SPARED, NUTRIENTS NEEDED

People ask me constantly about specific nutrients. They either want to know about the ones they think they might be missing, or those that they think they are getting in great abundance on their current dietary regimen. Remember that "more is not better" when it comes to nutrition. More exercise than you need will simply leave you sore, or make it impossible for you to exercise again for several days.

More sunlight than you require will burn you. Too much vitamin C will give you diarrhea. Too much iron will constipate you, and too much vitamin A is deadly. It's the same with every nutrient. Excess is just as problematic as deficiency. Aim for "just right" when it comes to nutrition.

The body sets up its own protective mechanisms to guarantee that too much of any given nutrient isn't assimilated. By tanning the skin, the body shields against excessive intake of vitamin D. Diarrhea prevents the overabsorption of vitamin C. If excessive quantities of vitamin B complex are consumed, they are eliminated via the urine. The body adapts to high intake levels of many nutrients by simply absorbing a lower percentage of them.

Iron and sunlight are two prime examples of this body-generated feature. The body also has the ability to adapt to changes in nutrient intake by adjusting the amounts eliminated, as it does with sodium. Too much protein, fat, or any other nutrient is never a good thing. Fortunately for us, becoming fat- or protein-deficient is almost impossible if we eat whole foods from the plant kingdom.

Calcium has become a nutrient about which many people are concerned. Calcium supplement sales are at an all-time high, as is calcium intake. Yet osteoporosis and other conditions of calcium deficiency are also at an all-time high, and rates are climbing steadily. Their cause is not lack of calcium consumption, but increased rates of calcium loss.

Calcium is lost when we get insufficient sunlight, and when we are inactive, especially when we place little or no strength demands upon our muscles and bones. The ingestion of dietary acids, such as the phosphoric acid in cola drinks, also causes calcium loss. Meat, dairy products, and most grains, are richer in acid minerals than they are in alkaline ones, whereas fruits and vegetables are richer in the alkaline minerals: potassium, calcium, magnesium, and sodium. When acidic foods dominate our diets, we lose calcium.

Hardening of the arteries, a condition in which calcium builds up on the inner arterial walls, is also on the rise. Apparently there is enough calcium in the blood for much of it to be deposited on the arterial walls. Striving to get enough calcium when it is being lost at such a rapid rate is something like trying to fill a bucket that has a huge hole in the bottom.

Absorption rates for many nutrients are controlled by the body at least to some degree, according to need. If your iron levels are high, for example, you will absorb a smaller amount of iron than if your iron levels are low.

As mentioned earlier, absorption rates are also affected by the dose of the nutrient to which we are exposed. The larger the dose, the smaller the percentage of absorption. Nutrient sparing is akin to recycling. When a cell dies, its contents are eventually dumped into the blood stream. At the site of the liver or the kidneys, nutrients that can be reused are sent back into circulation. Protein, most minerals, and many other nutrients are "spared" and reused in this manner, rather than being lost in the urine or neutralized in the liver.

Nevertheless, supplement salespeople will always have a new supplement to promote. Know that these substances simply are not necessary if one eats correctly. And if one does not eat correctly, supplements will not make up for the lack of nutrients and the influx of toxins. Getting enough of the nutrients we need to play with gusto and recover rapidly is easy. All we have to do is focus our diet so that it revolves around the consumption of copious quantities of whole, fresh, ripe, raw, organic fruits and vegetables.

HEALTHFUL LIVING BEGETS HEALTH

Taking Out the Garbage

Detoxification is a process that is going on within your body twenty-four hours per day, every day, as it always has been and always will be while you are alive. The liver and kidneys are the dominant organs of detoxification, though others can "pitch in" should they become overloaded with work. Detoxification equates with us getting well. When we detoxify via the eyes, ears, lungs, throat, nose, tongue, skin, and bowels, as well as the kidneys, liver, and other organs, we are getting well at an accelerated rate compared to the norm. Essentially, we are taking out more garbage than usual.

This represents an excessive amount of work for the body, and often leaves us feeling tired. Although we refer to this accelerated state of housecleaning as "being sick," it is actually a demonstration of

"When we detoxify via the eyes, ears, lungs, throat, nose, tongue, skin, and bowels, as well as the kidneys, liver, and other organs, we are getting well at an accelerated rate compared to the norm."

the body working perfectly, doing what it must according to its needs.

Internal cleanliness is not something that you can create through the consumption of a product. Cleaning is a bodily controlled action. The body will "clean house" in direct proportion to the degree that healthful substances, forces, influences, and conditions are provided and health-destroying ones are avoided. All efforts to intervene are ineffective, and most are counterproductive.

Health is the outcome of healthful living; symptoms are the result of compromises to healthful living. It's far more efficient and easy to keep the body clean in the first place than to make a mess of it and try to undo the damage later. Injuries are far less likely to occur and recovery is greatly enhanced when the body does not have to put excessive quantities of effort into its detoxification efforts.

Providing adequate sleep, fresh air, movement, pure water, moderate sunshine, and our natural foods goes a long way in reducing the amount of effort the body must direct to housecleaning.

One of the major premises of this book is that it is always better to correct a problem than to supplement it. All living organisms are self-cleansing, as well as self-monitoring, self-healing, and self-controlling in every way. Supply healthful conditions and your body will run itself as perfectly and as cleanly as is humanly possible.

Flushes, cleanses, nutritional support regimens, and various detoxification programs available on the market are not effective tools for reducing the toxic load of the body. They simply stimulate and irritate the body, resulting in an increased state of fatigue and enervation than before these programs were introduced.

Removing the cause of disease makes far more sense than treating the symptoms, and it is far easier to stay healthy than it is to get healthy. Still, there is a huge return on investment when you switch to healthier living habits. It's far more expensive in time, money and the way you feel to be sick than to be healthy. Your health is priceless.

Part 3—When Things Go Wrong

Things go wrong occasionally. In addition to making life challenging, mishaps make life interesting and give us opportunities to grow. In the immortal words of Elbert Hubbard, "Life is just one damned thing after another." In real life, compromise is inescapable: when mistakes happen, injuries occur, sleep is lost, training is interrupted, or nutritional goals are abandoned; dealing with the consequences can make you stronger.

9. Emergency Care and First Aid

Most of us are familiar with the standard guidelines for injury care. Should you get a small cut, you know to wash it, put antibacterial or antibiotic cream on it, bandage it, and leave it alone to heal. The following guidelines were designed to give you a basic template to follow when determining the level of care to give to an injury. Of course, every situation is unique, as is each person's perspective and assessment of the degree of damage done during any accident. Even if you follow the guidelines perfectly, some amount of personal thought and insight will have to be used when caring for every injury and each person that incurs it.

These basic guidelines can often be followed when handling most minor injuries. The protocols are useful to know, but judgment will likely play a part in dealing with every accident. Decisions need to be made about the nature of the wound. Is this shin injury a puncture, a scrape, or both? Does that wound need cleaning, or would cleaning it be counterproductive? Will a bandage do the job or does this cut require stitches? Should that gash be exposed to the air or should it be covered? And perhaps most important to consider: should professional medical assistance be sought, or is home care sufficient? Will I risk permanent impairment by not going to the doctor with this injury?

The following guidelines represent procedures that are to be used in a generic fashion only. They offer the basics in assessment, care, and follow-up, and should not be used to replace professional medical care. If you are not certain that you can handle the injury in front of you, it's a good idea to let the professionals take over. See Chapter 11 for an in-depth discussion of assessing injuries and knowing when to get professional aid.

PRICE'S RULES FOR EMERGENCY CARE

"Price's rules" for injury care are the classic interventional procedures. They are efficient and effective, and give both the person who is injured, and the person who is providing first aid, a satisfactory sense of thoroughness.

When creating generic injury care guidelines for mainstream use, the acronym "ICE" was formulated to remind people to care for most minor injuries through the use of "ice, compression, and elevation" on the affected part. This concept has been expanded upon over time. When someone realized that ceasing the activity which caused the injury was a sensible option, rest was added to the care procedures, resulting in a new acronym, "RICE."

As the need for follow-up care became more apparent due to the extended nature of many injuries, elastic wraps and orthopedic devices were developed, and an "S" for "support" was then added to the end of the acronym, making "RICE'S" the rule of thumb for injury care.

Our very first reaction to almost any injury is to hold the affected part. That is why the acronym eventually evolved to include a "P" for "pressure." Known as "Price's rules" today, this protocol highlights how to properly care for injuries from start to finish. Depending on the nature and degree of the injury, you may or may not utilize all of the elements of these "rules" before determining that care is completed.

PRESSURE

Applying pressure is almost an automatic response to injury. Hit your thumb with a hammer and you will likely grab the thumb with the other hand, and press on it firmly. You hold the thumb for a few moments, massage it gently, and then take a look at it. Once you realize there is no major visible injury, you wiggle your thumb a bit to ascertain that nothing is broken. If all seems well, you then go about your business, giving no more thought to this minor injury. You did the right thing. You applied pressure, and that was all you had to do in this case.

Normally, covering an open wound with your hand would also be appropriate. If the injury is mild but bleeding, applying light pressure will often stem the flow of blood. Should it be bleeding heavily, a stronger pressure from your hand can hold back the flow until more sophisticated measures can be taken. If there is a thorn, splinter, or other offending bit of debris in the wound, you will likely be able to feel and remove it with your hand before applying pressure. Applying pressure is our instinctual initial response to injury, and it is the correct response.

Completing the Brain-Body Circuit

Every cell of your body is in communication with every other cell via the brain. When you put your hand to an injured spot, your brain gets more messages about the injury and sets the appropriate responses into action. Feedback from the sensory nerves in your hand tells the brain almost everything it needs to know in order to bring about the desired healing effect. Touching your injury and applying pressure closes an electrical circuit in your body that hastens attention to the injured part.

"Applying pressure closes an electrical circuit in your body that hastens attention to the injured part."

REST

The second letter of Price's rules is "r," for rest. The wisest move is to rest any injured area. The amount of rest that is appropriate depends greatly upon the severity of the injury: the more severe the injury, the more rest is required. For many minor injuries, the application of pressure followed by a short period of rest is all that is required for complete recovery. Rest comes in many forms and degrees, as was discussed in Chapter 7, as well as in different fashions. Which fashion of rest to choose is a decision that only you can make.

If you have been raking leaves in the yard and begin to notice soreness on the palm of your hand, you may assume that you are about to get a blister. Rest can be achieved by switching hands, putting on gloves, holding the rake in a different manner, or by stopping for the day. If your back begins to hurt while you are playing badminton, you will have to decide if it is smarter to simply take a short rest from playing or if you are done for the day. In another scenario, you may get a cramp or turn an ankle in the middle of a run. Though you might stop completely to rest for a while, it is likely that you will walk the remainder of the distance to your home if possible. Rest in this case is walking rather than continuing your running.

Rest Is A Constructive Use of Your Time

Many people think of rest as a waste of time, or something that they should apologize for, if caught in the act. Some people think that resting equates with "doing nothing." Yet, rest is a time-honored pastime in many parts of the world. It *is* doing something. In the words of Dr. Wayne Pickering, "Rest is not doing nothing, it is an activity." The siesta has been around for a long time for a good reason.

Many people find that by adding a substantial rest in the middle of the day, they are much more productive and remain far healthier than when they try to push themselves through one long day. In fact, most people who lose energy and feel "run down" in the last few hours of their day find that they can totally avoid those feelings by resting at midday.

Review the section on rest in Chapter 7 to gain a fuller sense of how to apply rest in all situations relating to the treatment of injury. Physical, sensory, emotional, and physiological rest are all relevant when aiming to gain an edge on speedy recovery from injury. By giving rest the respect that it deserves in your overall health program, you will see that your health, fitness, and recovery all improve dramatically.

ICE

Long before there were drugs for controlling low- to mid-level pain, ice was used quite successfully for this somewhat questionable purpose. Ice has been used to reduce swelling as well, another function that is today being reexamined. Let's look at the negative aspects of these functions as well as the positive ones.

Pain Control

Ice slows most physiological processes in our body while reducing the speed and efficiency of nerve transmission, hence dulling our ability to sense pain. Ice should be used for about twenty minutes on and twenty minutes off intermittently, in order to keep certain types of acute pain at bearable levels.

When the ice comes off, however, nerves and blood vessels surge back into action (sometimes referred to as "Hunter's reaction") and the sensation of pain can become greater than if no ice had been used at all. Ice should generally be used only for pain control on injuries that are brand new, and certainly not for longer than one to two days.

Reduced Swelling and Blood Flow

No one likes to see the swelling that results after an injury, or to experience the discomfort that accompanies it. We are tempted to do what we can to reduce the swelling, and to keep it at a minimum. When ice is applied to any area of the body, blood and lymph flow to the area decreases, resulting in reduced swelling. Usually, when the swelling goes down, we feel better, at least emotionally.

Swelling serves many purposes in helping injuries to heal, however. With the initial swelling of an injury, many vital immune factors in blood and lymph are brought in abundance to the area of the wound, helping to minimize infection and promote healing. Swelling around an injured joint or broken bone effectively creates a splint that helps to stabilize the area.

The added stability allows for a minimal degree of mobility by the affected part, whereas otherwise none would be possible because of the pain generated around the unstable injury. By stabilizing joint or bone, swelling also helps accelerate and promote tissue repair because these injured areas heal more rapidly when they are kept in proximity to each other and not moved about.

Slowed Healing

Blood and lymph are important to the healing of any injury. Reducing the flow of these vital fluids can therefore be looked at in two ways. For the same reasons that swelling is reduced and nerve functions slowed when ice is applied, healing time is lengthened.

The processes of healing require nerve and blood function. Essentially, there is a trade-off: Pain reduction from the use of ice is offset by longer healing times. You may have less pain, but you are also likely to have the pain for longer. The decision remains up to the individual whether to use ice or not. I was an ardent proponent of icing for injury thirty years ago but today I avoid it. If the pain is so severe that it cannot be tolerated, I recommend professional medical intervention. Up until that point, I recommend that thought control and the remainder of Price's rules be utilized in order to minimize the intensity and duration of the pain, and to facilitate the healing responses of the body.

COMPRESSION

The application of compression to a wound aids the circulation and prevents pooling of blood; however, the pressure must be applied with great care and should be monitored closely. Too much pressure and the blood flow to the area can be completely cut off. This will result in increased pain, delayed healing, and, if left on long enough, can lead to the onset of gangrene.

Without enough compression—firm, light, pressure—the benefits described below will be completely lost. Compression can be achieved with a range of wrappings, from a small adhesive bandage to repetitive wrappings of cloth, elastic, or tape. Be sure to check on the pressure of the bandage every hour or so for the first twelve hours. If the swelling goes up or down, it can dramatically impact the effectiveness of the pressure bandage.

There are three primary goals to be achieved by using compression on an injury. First, the bandage helps to reestablish continuity between the damaged parts, holding them in close proximity to each other and keeping them relatively stable. Second, a pressure bandage protects the wound from outside airborne contamination and also from inadvertent damage by physical contact. Third, a properly applied pressure bandage will also spread the physical and physiological workload that is done by the body after an injury.

Physically it functions as a sort of "false skin" until the body can generate its own new skin and heal other affected parts. Also, by spreading the physiological workload, the bandage assists the body by allowing a greater area of cellular interaction with the injury. Swelling, contamination, debris from damaged cells, internal bleeding, and other physiological effects of injury are shared over a bigger area due to the proper application of a pressure bandage.

ELEVATION

Elevation is perhaps the smartest, most useful, and most underutilized of all of the steps of Price's rules. It is one that we would automatically use in nature, as even mild elevation provides almost instantaneous relief from the pressure caused by swelling and the pain of blood surging through an already engorged area. Elevating an injury effectively means positioning the wound or injured part so that it is physically higher than one's heart. A few inches' elevation will suffice in most cases. Too much elevation and it can become difficult for blood to reach the injury.

If you hurt your toe, for instance, and then decided to stay in a handstand, your toe would likely no longer hurt, but it also would not heal well. If the injured part begins to go cold, white, or black from lack of circulation, it is either because it has been elevated too high for too long, or the pressure bandage is too tight. Check all injuries periodically and make appropriate corrections.

One of the laws of hydraulics is that fluid cannot be compressed (at least not very much). When there is an injury, especially one accompanied by obvious swelling, all of the surrounding tissues are put under increased pressure. The skin stretches somewhat to accommodate the swelling, but even skin has limits. Taut skin means that with each beat of your heart, pressure in the area goes up dramatically. You can often feel each heartbeat as a painful, pounding throb.

This is because the sensory nerves in the area of the injury have also been damaged and they fire each time they are subjected to the increased pressure that accompanies the pulse. As soon as the injury is elevated to a location that is higher than the heart itself, the fluid pressure is dramatically reduced, as is the pain. Drainage of excess fluid is assisted by gravity, as is blood returning to the heart.

Pillows make one of the best elevation tools. They are soft, highly adjustable, disperse a load widely, and are not likely to add injury to the wound. Comfort is one of the most important factors when using elevation, as it is likely that the patient is going to have to remain in the chosen position for several hours or possibly even a day or two. If the injury is below the elbow or knee, be sure that the elbow or knee is positioned so that it is slightly bent, for comfort.

Weight should rest under the calf rather than the heel, and on the forearm rather than the hand. An excellent position for injuries to the shins, ankles, and feet is to lie on the floor supine (on one's back), as close to a bed or couch as possible, with calves resting upon the mattress of the bed or seat of the couch.

"Comfort is one of the most important factors when using elevation, as it is likely that the patient is going to have to remain in the chosen position for several hours or possibly even a day or two."

"Be very slow, methodical, and careful when changing position if the injured part is going to become lower than the heart."

Be very slow, methodical, and careful when changing position if the injured part is going to become lower than the heart. For instance, if you stand up to go to the bathroom, the change in pressure is extreme.

Not only is it likely to be quite painful if the change in position isn't achieved gradually, it is also possible that the injured person may lose consciousness. Fainting is often common shortly after an injury. Both shock and the radical change in blood distribution leave a person extremely vulnerable to blacking out. So go slowly when moving from a lying to a sitting position and pause again before moving slowly from sitting to standing and from standing to walking, making sure that the pain is manageable and that there is no feeling of light-headedness.

Depending upon the nature and intensity of the injury, gradually reduce the degree of elevation until it is comfortable to lie flat. As long as elevation provides relief, it is a useful positioning modality. Once it no longer provides relief, discontinue the use of elevation. You may find that as you resume normal activities, you are prone to some swelling around the affected area. In this case, elevation is the treatment of choice as it can always be used safely and effectively.

SUPPORT

There are many aspects to providing support for oneself during times of injury. In Price's rules, physical support is the typical focus. Braces, wraps, elastic clothing, stays, tape, and many homemade supports can be used as one begins the process of rehabilitating an injured body part back to health. Using such supportive devices on an interim phase of recovery is fine, but it is important to avoid their overuse.

As noted in the introduction to this book, "crutches cripple," and using a cane, brace, or any other support for too long, can mean developing dependence on it rather than freedom from it. Plan to gradually wean yourself from using and needing support devices by doing the required exercises or activities that will make them unnecessary. When the support becomes redundant, cast it to the side with glee and pride!

Many Types of Support

Supporting yourself during times of injury is crucial and can be done in many ways. Nutritional support is a significant factor, as was discussed in Chapter 8. Sleep, fresh air, sunlight and daylight, friendships, human touch, emotional poise, pure water, and many other lifestyle factors also play key roles in supporting one's recovery from injury. Each of these factors must be modified to meet our needs at any given time. When things are going well, it's relatively easy to follow any program. When times get challenging or stressful, however, it is common to veer off our chosen regimen.

Yet it is actually when times are challenging that we most benefit from staying focused on our chosen health routine, including food, sleep, and exercise habits.

Suppose, for example, that you have a goal of running in the London marathon. You have been training for months, and following a special diet. Then one day, just a few weeks before the event, you hurt your ankle severely.

You are upset about the injury and even more upset about the prospect of not running in the marathon. If you go to the local pub and have several beers and all the "wrong" foods, you may feel "better," but only because you have numbed your ability to process emotions. In fact, you have simply created a more acute emergency within your body via the alcohol (which acts as a poison, and must be dealt with as such by your body) and junk foods (which also must be processed laboriously and dealt with).

This behavior is not truly supportive of your highest goals. When it seems hardest to take excellent care of yourself, it is most essential. By doing so, you will truly be building your health.

THE ESSENTIAL FIRST-AID KIT

Like most things that require forethought, having a first-aid kit available when you need it won't happen unless you take specific steps to have one on hand. Since accidents happen unexpectedly, it is wise to follow the Boy Scouts' motto and "be prepared." Redundancy in first-aid kits is preferable to not having one at all. They do not have to be large or expensive to be effective. The bare essentials will do, as usually the same items are needed time and again. Don't get caught feeling silly because your first-aid kit hasn't been replenished with some common, yet essential item like an adhesive bandage, when needed.

CONTENTS

The following is a list of items recommended for your first-aid kit essentials, as well as some useful elective ones. The numbers in parentheses represent suggested quantities for each item. Lack of a number indicates that only one of the item is required.

Required Items

- Adhesive bandages — small (5), medium (10), large (5)
- Sterile gauze pads (10)
- Cotton balls or pads
- Sterile dressings: Variety of sizes
- Alcohol swabs (10)
- Elastic wrap bandage (2)
- Antiseptic wipes (10)
- Antibiotic cream, small tube
- Scissors, small, blunt
- Safety pins (10)
- Absorbent dressing (10)
- Triangular bandage

- Tweezers
- Surgical tape rolls: ½-inch and 1-inch

Optional Items

- Magnifying glass
- Athletic tape
- Calamine lotion
- Thermometer
- Surgical gloves
- Paper and pencil
- Flashlight
- Whistle
- Blanket
- Blood-pressure kit
- Glucometer

Location

Keep the first-aid kit easily (and quickly) accessible. For instance, if you have a large home and yard, keeping the first-aid kit in the attic is not a prime setup. You might even want to have two in such a situation and keep one in the house and one in the garage or shed. Keeping the first-aid kit near to where accidents are likely to happen is smart, as is keeping it out of the reach of children.

The kitchen, workshop, and play areas are ideal locations. There should also be a first-aid kit in every car, though most have none. A first-aid kit is like your wallet or purse; don't leave home without it. For specific travel trips, a kit can be tailored as needed. For example, my backpacking first-aid kit was extremely tiny and light, whereas the one I take to sporting events is "fully loaded" with a variety of options and plenty of extras.

Familiarity

It's smart to know what is in your first-aid kit and how to use it all. On a trip to Costa Rica once, I reviewed the first-aid kit and realized I had no idea how to use the snake-bite kit within it, and that in the unlikely event of a snake bite, I probably wouldn't have time to read the instructions. After I read the instructions carefully, I felt much better prepared. Become familiar with your kit's location, the items in it, and how to use each item.

"It's smart to know what is in your first-aid kit and how to use it all."

Updating

I once opened up an alcohol swab from my first-aid kit for a woman who needed to give herself an insulin injection, only to discover that the alcohol had evaporated and the swab had gone dry. The next three were from the same batch and had also all gone dry. Fortunately, I had plenty more, including eight that were still in good condition. I would have been embarrassed had they all been unusable! Keep in mind that tape also occasionally needs to be replaced. Check the contents of your first-aid kit(s) on a regular basis (yearly should be fine) to make sure that all of the contents are still functional—not outdated, dried up, rusty, or dysfunctional in any way—and replace any items as needed.

Stocking and Inventory List

A good time to check your inventory is when you are checking your first-aid kit for expired items. Either keep a running list of kit contents or count each item, and restock your kit as needed. Over time you will learn which items you wish to stock more of and which you need fewer of, but realize that first-aid needs are not easily predictable when used in small quantities. Hopefully, you will never need large quantities.

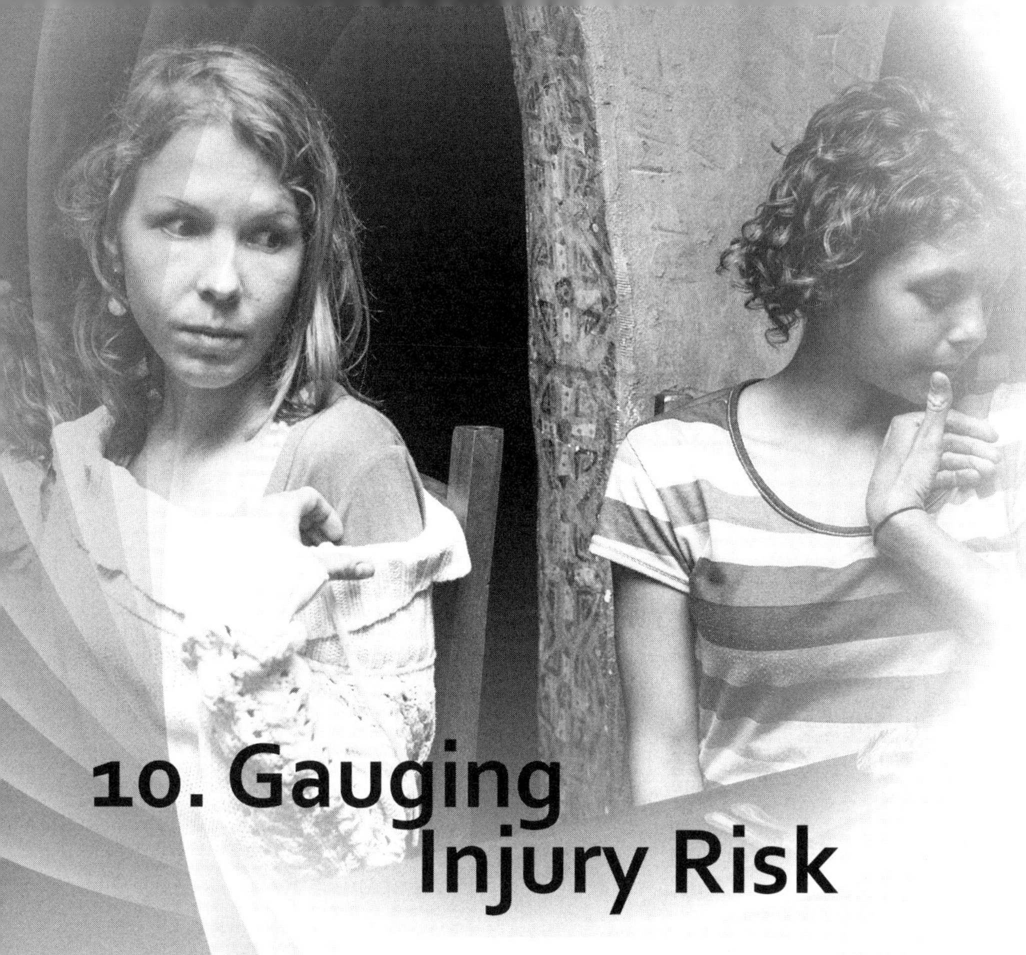

10. Gauging Injury Risk

A key to preventing injuries is knowing what types of injury you have a propensity for, based on the strengths and weaknesses inherent in your body. For example, if you know that you are prone to ankle sprains you can take special precautions against them: you can become more familiar with your ankles and their function, and you can choose activities that do not tend to aggravate or result in ankle sprains.

We must take our personal health into consideration when choosing fitness activities. When we do, we increase our chances of strengthening our overall health, and decrease our chances of inducing injury. An osteoporotic person might want to choose weightlifting to strengthen the bones, while avoiding full-contact karate, which could all too easily break a bone. An obese person would be wise to choose walking rather than running, and a person with arthritis will need to take his or her special joint needs and restrictions into consideration when choosing an activity.

WHO'S PRONE TO PARTICULAR INJURIES

When I was four years of age, we took my great aunt to the bus station. As the bus pulled away, I ran alongside it, enthusiastically waving goodbye to my aunt as she waved goodbye to me. While I was looking at her, I ran straight into a signpost, and a lump the size of an egg grew on my forehead to prove it. I learned a great lesson that day. Paying attention, and taking precautions when we can, will often keep us out of the path of injury.

Children

We must accept that children are prone to almost every conceivable injury. Fortunately, they can "get away with" most of these, as their joints tend to be far more flexible and their tissues far more pliable than those of adults. Children are also much more active than most adults, increasing the likelihood of their taking a tumble. Also, they have to learn their limits somehow, and this learning often occurs by pushing the limits of physics to the edge. In short, if you are in the care or vicinity of a child, keep your first-aid kit at the ready.

Women

In sports, women are prone to basically the same injuries as men, with the following exceptions.

- Women tend not to be as top-heavy as men; on average, they carry their center of gravity about four inches lower than men. This makes a woman more physically stable than a man and less likely to take a tumble. Women have an edge in sports such as skiing, surfing, and skating, where a low center of gravity is an advantage.
- Women are often more flexible than men but not as strong; hence they are more likely to incur joint injuries.
- Women must take special precautions against injuries to their breasts.

Seniors

Other than minor decreases in reaction time, balance, and connective tissue elasticity (muscles, tendons, and ligaments), seniors incur very few special risks of injury strictly as a result of their calendar years. Accumulated lifestyle habits do catch up with everyone, however, putting most seniors at risk because of the following:

- Loss of strength, which means slower reaction times, decreased joint stability, and a reduced ability to make up for poor balance, coordination, body mechanics, or judgment with sheer force.
- Generalized dehydration, which means that muscles and joints are more prone to injury.
- Lack of use due to sedentary lifestyle habits, which leads to the loss of functional abilities in daily chores that require muscular strength, muscular endurance, flexibility, neurological training, and cardiopulmonary fitness.

Loose-Jointed People

Some people are more flexible than others. People who are particularly loose-jointed, especially if they are not extremely strong, have a much greater chance of injuring their joints than of tearing muscles or breaking bones. Precautions must be taken, such as wearing supportive straps or using tape. Exercises to strengthen the structures that support the joint—muscles, tendons, and ligaments—are highly recommended.

Inflexible People

The inflexible person is not likely to experience joint injuries, but is much more prone to muscle tears and even to broken bones. Ideally, there should be a balance between strength and flexibility. Until that balance is achieved, it is wise for the inflexible person to put extra emphasis on flexibility training. The use of an extensive warm-up will prove useful in the interim until flexibility improves.

COMPLICATED HISTORIES CAN AFFECT OUR PRESENT HEALTH

The saying, "People are sicker than we give them credit for," has never been truer than it is in the 21st century. Many conditions that used to be considered diseases of aging such as diabetes, cancer, heart disease, stroke, chronic fatigue, and arthritis, among others, now earn the dubious distinction of requiring specialized children's wards in hospitals—and sometimes entire hospitals—in almost every major city. Unfortunately, the health conditions that have been plaguing adults now extend to our children.

"Unfortunately, the health conditions that have been plaguing adults now extend to our children."

Furthermore, it is extremely rare that a person with one condition, such as diabetes, doesn't also have at least one or two others. When a person has more than one condition at a time, it is referred to as a "complication." An estimated 95 percent of all adults in the Western world suffer from some degree of heart disease and over 75 percent also have the beginning stages of cancer.

With almost 40 percent of adults suffering from arthritis and almost half of the adult population showing diabetic or pre-diabetic symptoms, it is easy to see that a complicated health history is the norm these days rather than the exception. Over 80 percent of Americans reported taking prescription or over-the-counter medications last year to treat their health problems, and Europeans aren't far behind. When the following conditions are a part of one's health make-up, it is important to be aware of and take precautions as necessary to prevent injury.

Diabetes

Diabetics need to monitor their blood-sugar levels closely when performing any type of physical activity. They should become familiar with expected blood-sugar levels before, during, and after exercise, and compare these to their actual levels.

Chronic elevated blood-sugar levels of just 20 percent or more above normal leads to the destruction of eye, kidney, and nerve tissue. Dietary fat, and not sugar itself, is the prime culprit leading to sustained high blood-sugar levels, as fat in the bloodstream prevents sugar from exiting the blood, but not from entering.

Heart Disease

There are many forms of heart disease, all of which respond well to a low-fat (10 percent of total calories consumed) diet along with regular cardiopulmonary exercise done at an appropriate level of intensity. It is crucially important not to set off heart-disease symptoms while exercising, even when one's goal is to resolve heart disease. Care should be taken to be progress extremely gradually in all exercises undertaken. Slow and steady progress in most health pursuits beats any and all negative outcomes.

Hypertension

Hypertensive individuals need to take special care to avoid static contractions such as isometrics and all exercises that require straining. Proper breathing technique needs to be emphasized during all strength and muscular endurance activities, and even when stretching. Hypertension also responds well to a low-fat diet.

Arthritis

There are many types of arthritis, but for our general purposes it is only relevant to mention that people with arthritis need to be extremely careful not to injure themselves while exercising. They should choose activities that they can do painlessly, and safely. Arthritics tend to respond very well to flexibility exercises as well as to cardiopulmonary and other exercises that require high numbers of repetitions. Swimming is the classic exercise of choice for arthritics, and walking is also extremely valuable. If you are capable of rowing, cycling, or skating, these and any other cardiopulmonary exercises are also excellent choices.

Obesity

The strength demands placed on the obese person can make simply functioning in the home an effort. In obese people, the joints are under extreme stress—especially those of the hip, knee, ankle, and foot. One client told me that before she lost her excess weight, her main exercise challenge for the day was getting up from one chair in order to sit down in the next. Try going up a flight of stairs with an extra 140 pounds on your back in order to understand the immense strain an overweight person faces constantly. Walking and swimming are excellent exercises for the obese person.

The biggest risk of injury for obese people comes when they lose control of their own momentum. A slight misstep on stairs for a lightweight person will likely be a serious fall for a heavy person. Loss of balance can result in major injury. When moving rapidly, such as on a bicycle, a heavy person has tremendous momentum and must be overly cautious. Stopping often requires a much greater distance and more effort than one would think.

Respiratory Illness

The variety of respiratory illnesses makes it difficult to be specific about precautions without going into the intricacies of each condition; a requirement that is beyond the scope of this work. Asthma is likely the most common respiratory condition, however, and when one has asthma, it is vitally important not to set off an attack due to the exertions of exercise. Long and slow warm-ups are essential. Pushing the limits of breathlessness is not suggested unless you are extremely sure that this will not set off an asthma attack.

"Swimming, cycling, gentle rebounding, walking, and other non-jarring activities are the best choices if you have osteoporosis."

Osteoporosis

Osteoporosis is a condition whereby calcium is lost from the bones. The bones become weaker over time until they begin to fracture very easily and even spontaneously. Shocking or jarring force, such as when jumping or rapidly changing direction, can be sufficient to result in broken bones in someone with advanced osteoporosis. Full-contact sports are strictly contraindicated. Swimming, cycling, gentle rebounding, walking, and other non-jarring activities are the best choices if you have osteoporosis. Strength training is essential to stop, and hopefully reverse, the progression of this condition.

There are no health conditions for which healthful living is contraindicated. For all people, including those with the above-mentioned health conditions, healthful living includes a low-fat diet of approximately 80 percent of calories from carbohydrates via fruit, as well as sufficient sleep, water, fresh air, emotional poise, and proper exercise for our needs.

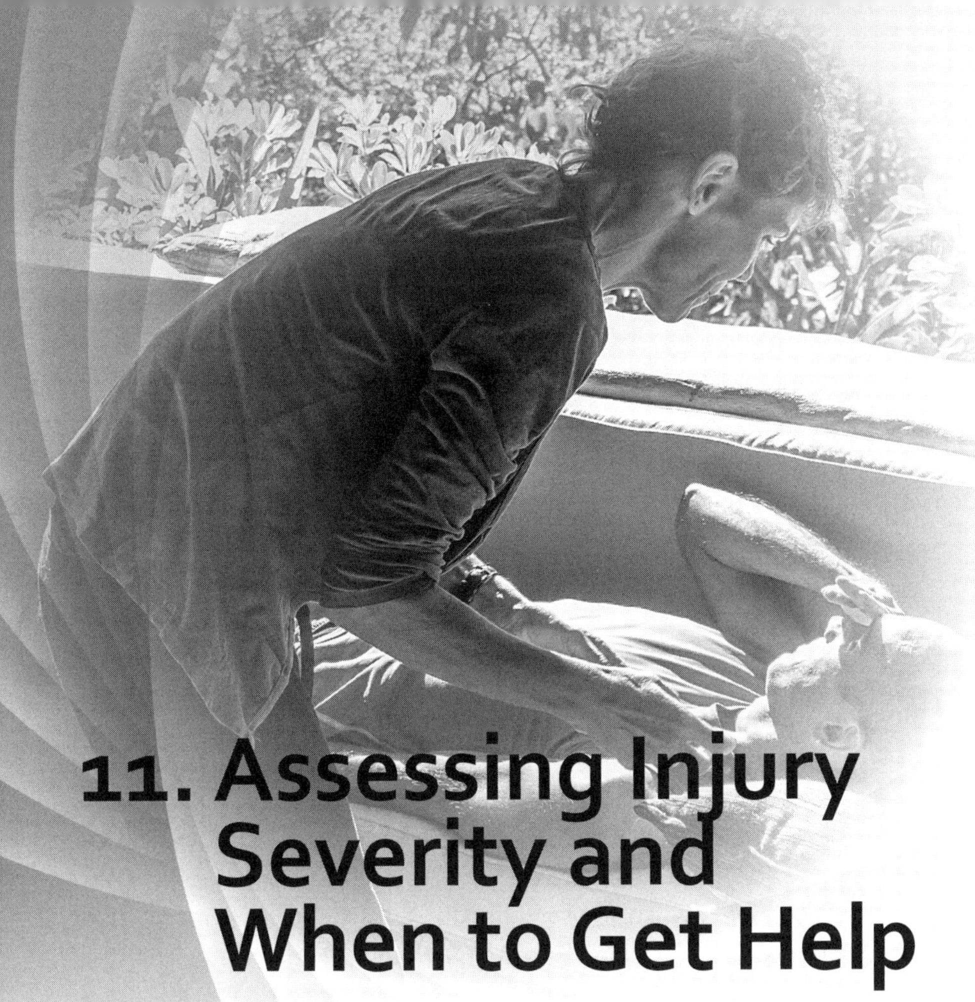

11. Assessing Injury Severity and When to Get Help

People's attitudes and perceptions about the severity of their injuries are unique. Some children take hard falls, get up, and don't even bother brushing themselves off before continuing with their play, while others cry from bumps that were imperceptible to anyone else. Even as adults, our response to an injury can be affected by who is watching or the activity we are involved in at the time. The expression "just a flesh wound" was taken to its hyperbolic extreme in the film Monty Python and the Holy Grail, *when the loss of a limb was considered a minor inconvenience.*

Of course, in real life, such a wound would be devastating. Yet, sometimes even minor injuries can be incapacitating, much to our dismay. For example, a runner or ballplayer with an injured big toe, may find it impossible to compete.

Most injuries require only minimal care, and can be dealt with at home. Of course, some injuries are so severe that there is no question about getting professional help, and often no choice.

ASSESSING INJURY SEVERITY

THE BASICS: RUBOR, DOLOR, CALOR, AND SWELLING

Over 2,000 years ago, human responses to injury were diligently chronicled. Four main categories of reaction were observed in injuries, even those that were expected to heal perfectly. Our physiological responses are no different today.

Rubor (Redness)

Rubor, or redness, almost always accompanies any physical injury, at least to a limited degree. The heightened metabolic activity that is always present after an injury is normal, and is reflected by redness in the area, but when redness spreads beyond the place of injury, it's time to pay attention.

Red streaks have serious implications, as they usually are a sign of blood poisoning. Streaking around a wound or infection, radiating towards the heart, should not be ignored. Seek medical attention immediately.

Dolor (Pain)

Dolor, the Latin word for "pain," is to be expected to some degree after any injury. When even the smallest nerve is damaged, pain is the result. While we would all like to escape the pain that accompanies injury, we would likely hurt ourselves far more frequently and severely were it absent.

The amount of pain experienced is not always indicative of the severity of an injury. Some minor injuries can be deceptively painful while there are many

"Generally speaking, pain and severity of injury go hand in hand."

serious injuries that elicit little pain. Usually, however, pain and severity of injury go hand in hand.

"The cessation of pain is a reliable indicator of when you're ready to resume physical activity."

No healthy person enjoys pain. There are many ways to manage pain, some of which are discussed in Chapter 9. However, reducing the amount of pain that we are capable of sensing, whether through the use of drugs or via "natural" intervention procedures, will invariably slow the healing response in all cases. It's always a good idea to respect your pain, live with it, and get it over with as quickly as possible by letting the body heal naturally. The cessation of pain is a reliable indicator of when you're ready to resume physical activity. Ignoring pain, or working through anything more than minimal amounts of discomfort, is never a healthy practice.

Calor (Heat)

The Latin word for heat is "calor." Localized heating of an injured area represents increased metabolic activity that almost always initially accompanies the healing of a wound. A useful skill to develop is the ability to discern by touch the difference between an injury that is warm (yet healing normally) from one that is disturbingly hot (and likely infected). An experienced hand can easily tell if there is cause for alarm.

"Watch and wait" is a reasonable approach to most minor injuries. If, however, the injury heats up alarmingly, or if the heat lasts for more than a few days, it may be time to get a professional opinion. When the heat is accompanied by rubor, dolor, and swelling, there is likely an infection. Such a situation should be watched closely. If it persists or worsens, seek medical attention.

Tumor (Swelling)

All irritation is followed by inflammation. The degree of irritation often is belied by the amount of inflammation. There are other factors, however, that can result in increased and often unexpected inflammation. Allergic responses, mineral or other nutritional imbalances, and infection, can all result in, accelerate, and increase the inflammation process.

There is a great temptation to try to reduce swelling whenever we see it. This is usually not the best option, however, as swelling serves many purposes within the body. For instance, in the case of joint injuries and broken bones, swelling around the involved area creates a cast-like effect that serves to stabilize the injury. Using anti-inflammatory drugs or agents will not only serve to slow the healing time, it will also reduce the stability created by the swelling.

An injury that remains swollen is receiving necessary attention from the body. Healing happens as rapidly as the body can produce it. While localized healing can be rushed through the use of medicinal drugs, it only serves to lower the vitality of the remainder of the body. Just as you trust your body to keep your heart beating and liver functioning, it is important to trust in the body's self-healing powers too. By respecting your body's agenda, and letting healing happen naturally at your body's chosen speed, you give yourself the opportunity to heal more efficiently and completely.

INJURIES WE MIGHT IGNORE TO KEEP PLAYING

Most injuries can simply be ignored. Minor bumps, scratches, twists, pulls, tweaks, cuts, grazes, and the like are so common, and so easily dealt with, that they barely warrant a blip on our radar. If you are hurt in one of these ways while playing a game, very often there is no need to interrupt it in order to get treatment. If continuing your game feels more important to you than tending to your injury, you're probably fine doing so. Of course, you have nothing to prove in this area, and you are well within your rights by taking time to fully examine even the most minor of injuries. Fortunately, most of our miscues are minor ones.

Blood

The sight of blood is worthy of attention. The basic question to ask when you see your blood coming from your injury is, "Will this stop bleeding on its own?" If a wound is so minor that it has already stopped bleeding, or you believe it will stop bleeding without further care, you can probably just ignore the injury and continue having fun.

Pain

Pain is a relative term that can only be measured subjectively. When newly injured, ask yourself to rate your pain level from one to ten, with ten being the highest. If the answer is a one or two, keep right on playing. If the pain reaches a three, you may want to consider the possibility that you have hurt yourself more seriously than you initially thought.

STOP, ASSESS, AND TREAT IF NEEDED, AND RESUME

There are times when injury requires immediate care but nothing more. When the contact is severe enough to warrant cleaning, bandaging, support, or other care, take the time to administer it. Usually after the application of basic first aid to such an injury, most people can go right back to the game without missing a beat.

Minor Contact

Even most noncontact sports lead to at least some casual contact, and sometimes that physical contact brings about injury. When one person runs into another, it is always a good idea to check in with yourself (or your teammate if you did the bumping) and make sure that no damage was done. If there is no blood, and the pain level is low, there is very little to do other than continue playing.

Keep in mind that even in situations where you ignore the injury and continue playing, it is a good bet to check out the site of the wound several more times during the course of the day. Sometimes our ability to recognize the serious nature of an injury is dulled by the amount of adrenaline we've been producing in the heat of play. Sometimes a seemingly minor hit can bring about a serious bruise later in the day.

You would be smart to keep a watch on all injuries, no matter how small or minor, and track their progress as they heal.

Shook-Up

An unexpected collision, a fall, a misstep, or even a hard landing can leave you shaken. After any such accident, it is wise to take time to thoroughly assess the damage done. If there is none, or if the injury is minor, it is perfectly acceptable to get right back into your training. Picture most children's responses after unexpectedly falling down: they pick themselves up, dust themselves off, check for obvious signs of injury, and—finding none—resume play.

Dazed but Not Confused

I was at the bottom of a very long ski run, cautiously approaching the line to get back onto the ski lift. I was going slowly, being careful to look out for beginners or other folks who might be having trouble when—POW!—a skier who was totally out of control crashed into me from behind and to the side, knocking me completely off of my skis. It was an absolute surprise, and because the skier was much bigger than I was, a very hard impact that really shook me up. The guy didn't even say, "I'm sorry." But I did my damage assessment, realized I was OK, put my skis back on, and got back in line. Should you fall off your bicycle, get hit by a thrown ball, or accidentally run into someone while playing, you might be momentarily dazed. As long as you remain conscious, know exactly who and where you are, and are showing no other signs of injury or confusion, you are probably best to simply continue on as if nothing had happened.

MINOR FIRST AID

It's a good idea to have at least a rudimentary first-aid kit on hand any time a group of people gather for sport. The simplest kit consisting of a few bandages, a wrap, and some tape will do. Carrying an adhesive bandage in your wallet would qualify as

"You would be smart to keep a watch on all injuries, no matter how small or minor, and track their progress as they heal."

the minimum that you could do without making any serious allowance for injury.

Adhesive Bandages

Adhesive bandages have come a long way in the last few years. They stay on better than they used to. They don't hurt as much as they used to when removing them. There are even waterproof adhesive bandages available now that will stay on under conditions of heavy perspiration, rain, and even while swimming. There are adhesive bandages that provide extra padding, extra absorbency, and even some with antibacterial medicines already saturated into the padding. Adhesive bandages come in a wide variety of sizes to meet practically every need, and a wide variety of colors, including clear, so as to be as unobtrusive as possible. A simple adhesive bandage can staunch the flow of blood from most wounds amazingly well.

In less than one minute's time after an injury, the wound can be assessed, cleaned, and bandaged. You can be back on the playing field, safe, and ready to go without spilling another drop of blood, with your wound fully protected.

Adhesive Bandages for Blisters

The development of a blister does not have to mean the end of the day's play any longer. An entirely new type of adhesive bandage has been developed that is designed to cover tender blisters, and it does an incredibly good job. These bandages have a gel padding in the cloth area that is to directly cover the wound. The gel padding protects the blister so well that it is actually difficult to tell if it is there at all. Once applied, the top of the bandage provides a slick, frictionless surface for socks or other clothing to slide on, so that more or deeper blisters do not develop in the area covered by the adhesive bandage.

Protective adhesive bandages really work well, and can mean the difference between continuing or quitting your activity in many instances. Since blisters often require a week or more to fully heal, a well-applied adhesive bandage can make a huge difference in your participation in fitness activities. When I developed a blister on the first day of a hiking trip, I put on an adhesive bandage and hiked the rest of the trip—eight more days—without a single problem.

Wraps

There are several different designs of wraps that can be utilized "on the fly" to enable someone to continue playing safely after receiving a mild injury. There are elasticized cloth bandages of varying widths and lengths that can be quickly applied and secured. There are also several types of rubber and cloth wraps that close with a tie or Velcro. There is even an elasticized gauze tape, Elastikon, that can be applied on its own, under tape, or over cloth. Any of these wraps will provide quick protection and support to a minor injury so that an enthusiastic player can safely continue the activities of the day.

See Chapter 9 for further discussion of first-aid kit supplies to keep readily available.

WHERE TO DRAW THE LINE

How Important Is It?

There is a limit to the degree of injury that can be safely ignored in the name of continuing the game. I do not recommend that anyone ever ignore serious injuries in order to continue playing. A line must be drawn, and I recommend drawing it conservatively, on the side of caution. The game isn't ultimately that important; it will likely go on without you, and there will always be another game, another time.

Do You Make Your Living Doing This?

If you do not make your living playing sports, you should not feel any compunction to continue playing if you have been hurt badly enough to question whether you should. Athletes who do make their living at sports are smart enough to know that they will be better respected and have a longer career if they stop to take good care of themselves, rather than press on and risk compounding their injury unnecessarily. Pros willingly pull themselves out of games, knowing that there is always tomorrow. Knowing when to play on, and when to quit for the day, is one of the most important decisions you can make.

STOP, TREAT, AND REST

As disappointing as it can be, there are times when cutting your activity short due to injury is simply the right thing to do. (This is not the same as being hurt so badly that you have no choice but to stop activity.) Following are some guidelines for recognizing when you would be best to simply call it a day.

Major Contact

Whether accidental or as an integral part of the game, occasionally we experience a major contact with other people, stationary objects, and sometimes even with the ground. In these instances, it is especially beneficial to take your time and methodically assess the damage. You may have hurt yourself in more than one place. Scan your body mentally first, then visually, then tactilely. The harder the hit, the more important it is that you are thorough in your evaluation.

Smart Is As Smart Does

Accidents happen; it's just a fact of life. Sometimes though, in the excitement of the moment, you can make unwise decisions when initially hurt. When you are injured, try to assess the damage with objective eyes and not the eyes of someone who was in the middle of an exciting, refreshing, and possibly important session or game. See the injury through the eyes of someone who truly has your best interests at heart. Attempt to separate yourself from the moment and treat the injury as part of the bigger picture that makes up the whole of your life.

Knowing Is Not Enough, Practice What You Preach

Advising someone else to rest is often far easier than resting ourselves. (It is relatively easy to hand out good advice, but following it ourselves is another matter.) Injuries need not be compounded for any reason. When you know it is time to stop because of an injury—stop! It may be the smartest training move you will ever make.

INJURIES IN-DEPTH

BRUISES: JOINT, BONE, AND MUSCLE CRAMPS

We all take our share of bumps and bruises. Some are more serious than others, but all of them deserve at least some initial attention, even if they never get a second thought. The severity of a bruise that results from injury is not solely determined by the intensity of the impact. If a bruise is sufficiently forceful to result in broken capillaries, there will be internal bleeding.

The blood is visible under the skin as it dissipates through the tissues until it is picked up by the lymphatic system. This is what gives bruises the black-and-blue, purple, and brown-and-yellow colors that we see following many trauma injuries.

Mineral and Nutritional Imbalances

Nutrition, along with several other lifestyle factors such as obtaining sufficient vitamin D from exposure to the sun, play a huge role in the creation of a durable body that can stand up to the vagaries of strenuous exercise,. If you find black-and-blue marks on yourself and you don't know where they came from, it is very likely that you are not consuming sufficient fruit. People who bruise extremely easily typically consume insufficient quantities of fresh fruit and the capillary fragility factor it contains.

The vitamin C complex is composed of many distinct parts: vitamin C, ascorbic acid, rutin, hesperidin, and capillary fragility factor, to name a few. Capillary fragility factor is so named because an insufficient amount of this vital nutrient results in tiny blood vessels (capillaries) becoming frail and bleeding extremely easily. Capillary fragility factor is found primarily in fresh fruit, though it is also found in peppers and a few other vegetables.

To build the levels of capillary fragility factor up to acceptable levels can take months, however, so do not be disappointed if results are not instantaneous. Smoking, pollution, and many other stresses, substantially increase one's need for capillary fragility factor and the entire vitamin C complex.

The primary extracellular mineral is sodium and the primary

intracellular mineral is potassium. Sodium deficiency is almost unheard of, whereas excess of this mineral is a common problem. Potassium deficiency, on the other hand, is quite common among people on the standard American diet.

"Sodium deficiency is almost unheard of, whereas excess of this mineral is a common problem."

Fruit is a wonderful source of potassium and vegetables supply us with all the sodium we need. Of course, fruits and vegetables need to be predominant in the diet in order for them to supply these nutrients in sufficient quantities. The ratio of potassium to sodium, when fruits and vegetables dominate the diet, comes out almost perfectly, regardless of the fresh fruits or vegetables that are chosen.

Hyaline Cartilage Damage

The ends of your bones are covered with a hard, glossy, almost glass-like cartilage. Called hyaline cartilage, it keeps friction to a minimum when a joint goes into action. There are no nerve endings that extend into this cartilage.

Because the amount of nerve tissue in an area directly affects the rate of healing after injury, it is easy to understand that damage to the hyaline cartilage can be extremely slow to heal. Bruising the cartilage creates an injury that is much like what happens when you strike safety glass with a crushing blow—it fractures into pieces, but largely stays intact.

If you stub your toe severely enough, it's likely that this sort of damage to the hyaline cartilage will occur. Be patient; it will usually heal in time.

Bone Bruises

Bone bruises are not very different from fractures in terms of how they heal. A severe bruise can take four to eight weeks to heal. You will likely need a week or more of recovery for even a mild bone bruise.

Once you understand that the body must create and lay into place entirely new bone cells to replace the damaged ones, it is easier to appreciate the time element involved in healing from bone injuries. Understanding what a realistic timeframe for healing is likely to be will help athletes set realistic recovery and training goals. Usually, we underestimate how long recovery truly takes.

Cramps

Muscle cramps can range in severity from minor inconvenience to major problem. There are many causes of muscle cramps. Nutritional imbalances, especially concerning the minerals sodium, potassium, and calcium, often are the cause of cramps. Cramps will often relax if steady pressure is applied to the belly (middle) of the involved muscle for five to fifteen seconds.

A cramp can also occur if a muscle is not getting sufficient blood supply to meet its immediate needs. The likelihood of cramping is why eating a heavy meal, or foods that are slow to digest, is not recommended before engaging in fitness activities.

Digestion and physical exertion both require large quantities of blood. As there is not sufficient blood available to perform both activities at once, either digestion, or the physical activity, will be compromised. Cramps are not usually dangerous, unless they occur while you are in the water. This is why swimming is not recommended for at least thirty minutes, or longer, after eating a meal.

CUTS: NONBLEEDING CUTS, SHARP CUTS, BLISTERS, AND ABRASIONS

There are seemingly no end to the variety of ways in which we can manage to hurt ourselves. In the world of fitness activities, opportunities to break the skin are abundant. Collisions with other people, friction from equipment, falls, and many other accidents, can easily lead to punctures, blisters, scrapes, lacerations, and gaping, bleeding wounds.

Seeing blood is often like seeing oil under the car in the garage: unexpected and potentially cause for concern. And since we are not used to seeing our own blood, losing just a small amount can be frightening. Nevertheless, bleeding used to be a fact of life in many sports. Blood was borne like a badge of courage. However, in today's contagion-shy world, an athlete with even the smallest amount of blood visible will be pulled from the competition and treated, at least sufficiently to quell the bleeding. Fortunately, with the precautions taken in today's sports, most events go from start to finish without producing so much as one drop of blood.

Nonbleeding Cuts

It's possible to damage the skin without producing an overt bleed. Minor injuries, surface wounds, cuts where the skin flap can be successfully replaced, and even certain abrasions and blisters, will not tend to bleed. They must still be dealt with as injuries, however, and should not be taken too lightly or dismissed altogether simply because they are not bleeding. Treatment includes thorough washing of the area and the application of a supportive bandage that completely covers the wound and all sensitive areas around it.

Some cuts and scrapes are slow to bleed because the capillaries that normally would ooze blood from the wound have been damaged in such a way that they are blocked off. Depending upon the number and degree of damaged capillaries, this type of bleeding can be difficult to stop, once it finally starts. By putting pressure on the wound, and covering it with absorptive material, you encourage the formation of a clot that will eventually form a scab.

If no surface blood vessels—or at least no particularly large ones—are damaged, it is possible that some injuries will not bleed at all. Puncture wounds, for example, often do not bleed externally, but can be quite severe.

"A surface injury that looks relatively clean and bleeds freely is far less likely to become infected than one that looks clean but is a nonbleeding puncture wound."

There is danger of internal bleeding and also of infection. When a wound is quick to bleed, the blood often helps to carry away any contaminants to which the body may have been exposed from the injury. A surface injury that looks relatively clean and bleeds freely is far less likely to become infected than one that looks clean but is a nonbleeding puncture wound.

Sharp Cuts

In a typical cut, the two surfaces are jagged, both on a visible as well as a microscopic scale. The jagged edges fit into each other and lock together, much like puzzle pieces. The blood that is caught in this "tight fit" forms a thin film that adheres to both sides of the wound, begins to clot, and forms a scab. Healing is then relatively rapid: once the scab forms, new cells are laid underneath it that will essentially "knit" the two sides of the wound together.

Extremely sharp objects can cut your skin so cleanly that the two surfaces of the wound do not want to adhere to each other again. Blood can't seem to get a grip on these smooth surfaces either, and so is slow to clot. This is why it is sometimes very difficult to get razor cuts, paper cuts, glass cuts, and some injuries in sport to stop bleeding. By applying pressure and elevating the affected part higher than the heart, you can reduce blood flow to the area and encourage clotting and scab formation.

Blisters and Rips

Blisters typically form on the hands or feet when you are performing a repetitive activity that you are not used to. For instance, perhaps one of the most common causes of blisters each fall is raking leaves. A pair of shoes that fit improperly will also quickly lead to blisters.

As the friction irritates the skin, the surface layer will dislodge from the underlying layers. Protective gear can go a long way toward discouraging blisters from forming. For example, in the beginning of baseball season, when batters are not used to holding the bat, the use of batting gloves will prevent blister formation. For many sports, doubling socks prevents blisters: the socks slide against each other rather than rubbing against the skin.

Rips form in much the same way as blisters. Like blisters, they are due to a combination of pressure coupled with rubbing. In the case of blisters, the pressure is usually much less than in the case of a rip, and the blister takes much longer to form. A rip will often occur long before there is any warning of blister formation.

I once watched a young boy swinging hand over hand across a set of bars at a playground. There were about 20 bars in total, and he really wanted to make it the entire way across. He got about 12 bars across and then dropped to the ground and looked at his hands. A patch of skin about the size of a quarter had ripped from one palm. The boy stared at his hand in seeming disbelief; he likely had never seen such a thing before. The pain had not yet set in, but an injury encompassing that much surface area was going to cause plenty of throbbing for a few hours. His palm would likely remain sensitive for almost two weeks before completely healing. Of course, had he been wearing gloves there would have been no injury at all.

Gymnasts are prone to rips on their hands as they rotate around the bars, rings, and pommels. However, if you look closely, you will notice that the gymnasts use special protective gloves, known as "grips," to keep their palms safe.

Care for such injuries is fairly simple. For blisters, if you can resist opening them, they will heal well on their own. The pocket of "water" that forms under the skin within the blister acts as cushioning for the delicate skin underneath, padding it from any future injury. If the skin breaks and the water leaks out, try to leave the remaining top skin intact and in place. The skin flap will protect the underlying skin and eventually fall off of its own accord. Rips should be kept covered and well-protected from use or reinjury. They are prone to drying and cracking—painful occurrences that delay healing.

"If you can resist opening blisters, they will heal well on their own."

Almost any form of moisturizer works well on the delicate skin under the rip, but you want to be sure not to use creams that have irritants in them, as it will burn the new skin. Creams with alcohol will dry the area more than moisturize it. Pure cocoa butter, shea butter, jojoba oil, or even plain vegetable oil, will do a fine job of keeping the skin moist so that it doesn't dry and crack.

Abrasions

Abrasions are similar to rips in that they are usually caused under substantial pressure coupled with friction while sliding on a rough surface. Whereas a rip "only" takes off the outer layers of skin, abrasions are deeper. The depth of an abrasion can range from just deeper than the skin (sometimes referred to as a "strawberry" because of the color pattern that results) to quite deep.

As long as "abrasive" force is applied, the resulting injury is technically an abrasion. Usually if the injury goes considerably deeper than the skin, even it is formed from abrasive forces, it will be treated and referred to as an injury other than abrasion. We therefore tend to think of abrasions as being primarily surface injuries.

Abrasions are problematic because they often encompass a great deal of surfacc area. This tends to make for a very long healing time, as skin is repaired from the edges of a wound inward towards the center. Directly under the skin is a rich bed of capillaries and accompanying lymphatic vessels.

When large areas of these vessels are damaged, wounds are exposed and vulnerable to outside contamination. Also, abrasion injuries tend to weep a great deal because it takes a long time for the lymphatic vessels to mend. Forearms, shoulders, hips, and knees are common areas that are susceptible to abrasion injuries. Such wounds should be cleaned well, as the usual cause of the abrasion is contact with asphalt, gravel, or artificial turf, all of which tend to be quite dirty. Once cleaned, abrasions should be kept covered, with bandaging changed as needed, until a solid and complete scab forms.

Skin Integrity

We have covered the treatment of many types of damage that can happen to the skin. The amount of surface area involved, the depth of the wound, and the amount of bleeding when skin is damaged, is critical in determining the recovery time. Generally, smaller wounds heal more rapidly, unless they are also deep wounds. The skin has many layers, hence many variations of injury are possible. Every conceivable injury to bone, tissue, and skin, is not covered in these pages, just the most common ones.

When the integrity of the skin is broken, you have a completely different injury than when the skin remains intact. The skin offers a barrier of protection from the outside world. Infectious agents, contaminants, toxins, and plain debris, are kept out of the body by the skin. Breaks in the skin should not be taken lightly. All damage to the skin should be washed thoroughly. If warranted, the damaged skin should be covered, at least until the body can create a scab. Wounds to the skin should be examined regularly to check for signs of infection, swelling, pus, or any unexpected abnormality of healing.

TEARS: SPRAINS AND STRAINS

The muscles, tendons, and ligaments of the body are graced with a degree of elasticity. Muscles are the most elastic, ligaments the least. One of the results of a warm-up is that this elasticity increases. When these tissues are stretched beyond their elastic limits, however, fibers within them fray and tear in a manner similar to that of a piece of rope. If the jolt is sudden and severe enough, it is possible to completely snap the muscle, tendon, or ligament into two pieces. Should that happen, you have a serious injury to heal from.

Fortunately, such an injury is relatively unusual. Minor tearing is much more common. The amount or degree of tearing, and the type of tissue involved, will dictate appropriate care for the injury, but primarily, forced rest is the treatment of choice. Once fitness activities for the injured part can be resumed, appropriate flexibility and strength training should also be included as part of the rehabilitation.

Sprains: Acute and Chronic

Each new sprain is an *acute* injury at the time it happens and for the next several days. But if you sprain your ankle repeatedly, it has become a *chronic* problem. Sprains refer to injuries of the ligaments, in which they are stretched beyond their elastic limits. Other tissues, including blood, lymphatic vessels, and even the neighboring bones are often damaged as well in a sprain.

The classic sprain occurs to the lateral (outside) portion of the ankle. There are more ligaments supporting the medial (inside) portion of the ankle than the lateral. Typically the range of motion is also greater on the lateral portion of the ankle, making for more mobility when turning the foot inward (inversion) as compared to outward (eversion). Thus, the likelihood of spraining the ankle into hyperinversion is far greater than that of spraining it in favor of eversion. A hypereversion sprain is almost an unknown event.

Each time a joint is stretched to the point of incurring a sprain, the ligament damage results in a ligament that is just a little bit longer healed than it was prior to the sprain; a condition often referred to as "ligament laxity." If you sprain an ankle once or twice a year for several years, for example, the ligament laxity can become so extreme that the ankle joint becomes noticeably unstable and quite prone to future sprains. The sprains may become increasingly severe as well, and eventually result in dislocations of the ankle. Appropriate physical therapy would include learning postural and walking skills to reduce the likelihood of future sprains by bringing more weight through the big toe instead of on the outside toe. Strengthening the musculature that everts the foot is also useful, as with increased strength there is improved stability, as well as faster reactions.

People with a chronic tendency toward sprains need to take appropriate precautions before engaging in physical activities. They must assess the likelihood of a sprain occurring during the considered activity. They must be willing to wear the appropriate protective gear; use the necessary tape, brace, or support; or simply say, "I think I am going to pass on basketball today—I tend to sprain my ankle whenever I play."

When sprains become severe enough, bones will hit against bones, resulting in potentially severe bruises. Repeated bruising of bone is one way to develop arthritis. Severe sprains are also likely to result in internal hemorrhages and lymphatic vessel tears. Arthritic, swollen, black-and-blue, weak, and tender joints are no fun. Strengthen weak joints, learn improved body mechanics, and wear the appropriate protection in order to put sprain injuries forever in your past.

Strains: Mild, Moderate, and Severe

Strain injuries typically occur to muscle or tendon fibers. They can occur in the main part of the muscle (the "belly"), where the muscle dovetails with the tendon (musculo-tendinous junction), in the tendon itself, or, least likely, near the point where the tendon attaches to the bone.

The severity of a strain is primarily gauged by the time required for the injury to heal. Quantities of tissue damaged, and the location of the strain, play major roles in making this determination. Typically, a mild muscle strain will heal in three days or less. A moderate strain will heal in one to two weeks. Moderate strains often occur at the musculo-tendinous junction.

Severe strains can take from several months, to a year, to heal fully. These chronic strains are sometimes referred to as tendonitis, or, if they occur at the junction of tendon and bone, are typically named by their location. Such is the case with lateral epicondylitis, commonly referred to as tennis elbow. In all strain injuries, the primary requirement for healing is simply the provision of sufficient rest to the affected parts.

CAN'T SHAKE IT OFF?

Often an injury that seems pretty bad at the moment of contact can be reduced to almost nothing in less than a minute or two of walking, moving, and stretching. The expression, "shake it off" is to be taken quite literally, as we can often "shake off" injury almost as effectively as a duck can shake water off its back. When we are hit, blood flow and nerve function to the area can be adversely affected, and on occasion, simply shaking the affected part will bring about a correction in the blood or nerve dysfunction. Sometimes it isn't that simple. Fortunately, professional help is almost always available.

MAJOR INJURIES AND WHEN TO GET PROFESSIONAL HELP

In almost every field of athletic endeavor there is some risk involved. Life itself is risky business for that matter, whether you leave your home or not. Fortunately, we have created a wide assortment of guards that remain available in the case that help is needed. On any ski mountain, the ski patrol is usually evident. Ski patrollers promote safe skiing, but also are there to help you should you need it. Every public swimming pool and many beaches have lifeguards. They pretty much have an all-or-nothing type of job. Usually there is nothing to do except remind people to act responsibly.

But when a lifeguard is needed, it is usually a life-or-death situation that requires a rapid, clear-headed response. Paramedics are on-call all hours of the day. In many communities, their response time to calls for help is measured in seconds, like firefighters. Having this type of help available is truly a blessing, and should not be taken for granted.

Athletic events of all types and at all levels of proficiency should have provisions for administering first aid. Learning the skills required to assist someone in an emergency is always a good idea, as you never know when it will come in handy. "Hi, my name is ________, and I am here to help you," are the best words an accident victim can ever hear. Too many people die with others standing idly by, watching but not knowing what to do. Once you have been helped by a lifeguard, ski patroller, paramedic, or the like, you will never take their services for granted again.

There is a certain temptation to try to do it all yourself, to be the most giving, and even to take the limelight when it comes to caring for someone with an injury. Yet recognizing that professional help is needed, and obtaining it, is one of the smartest moves that any caregiver can make. Sometimes, it is obvious that help is needed and sometimes the decision is not as obvious. With any injury whose severity makes you feel uncertain or insecure about caring for it on your own, seek medical assistance.

POLAR MINDSETS REGARDING PROFESSIONAL ASSISTANCE

There are two schools of thought about going to the doctor for any and every injury. Some folks feel that is what the doctors are there for. They feel entitled to the health care that they pay for, and that seeking professional help is the right way to go. On the other hand, there are many people who feel that the more they can take care of themselves, the better off they are. They do all they can to stay away from doctors. They wield their first-aid kits with confidence, and are willing to take some risks in terms of self-treatment, rather than take the risks of being treated by the medics.

There is no right or wrong side of this issue; it is totally about personal preference. Even the available data that might help you decide if you should go to the doctor is terribly unclear.

We know from recent statistics that medical error is the number one leading cause of death in the United States. This makes it appear that going to the doctor is very risky business indeed. Yet we don't know how many people are saved exactly because they went to the doctor when they did. It's easy to badmouth doctors, but would anyone really want to take their job? Every situation is an emergency, every patient has a complicated history, every situation is pressed for time, and decisions must be made and made correctly, or they stand to lose a patient.

Again, it is not that one way is right and the other is wrong. This is simply a matter of preference. Still, when it comes to caring for emergencies, it is prudent to let the doctors do their job. After all, they do have the benefit of experience. The following situations are ones where it is unquestionably a smart move to seek professional medical help.

UNCONTROLLABLE BLEEDING

When an injury initially occurs, there is nothing to stop the bleeding. The body acts quickly, however, to stem the flow of blood. The ends of the damaged vessels almost immediately contract, reducing and sometimes stopping blood leakage. The blood vessels in the vicinity of the damage constrict, further reducing blood flow to the area. Once blood actually exits from the damaged vessel, factors within the blood itself (platelets, fibrinogen, serum, antibodies, red blood cells, and specific "clotting factors") begin the formation of a clot. This is often sufficient to plug the hole in the vessel.

Much of the capillary damage will heal itself, but if the body does not stem its own blood flow, further treatment options are available. The pressure and support provided by the application of absorbent bandages and an adhesive covering will usually do the job. If dark red blood (an indication of damage to a vein) is still oozing from a wound after the injury has been cleaned and bandaged, treatment can be applied in the form of direct pressure and elevation. The use of all of these techniques almost always yields successful results when you are attempting to control and stop an injury from bleeding.

The average person has about ten pints of blood in total. To lose even a little blood usually seems like a lot, since we are generally excessively aware of any loss of blood. Still, we can lose a pint, the amount donated when we give blood, without showing any overt symptoms. By the time three pints of blood are lost, however, there will be serious compromise to our ability to function. If a severe wound does not stop bleeding, all local blood vessels will constrict in order to conserve blood to the brain and vital organs. This usually denotes the onset of the condition known as shock, recognized by the clammy pale appearance of the skin caused by the diverting of blood, coupled with sweating.

If there is uncontrollable bleeding with massive quantities of blood lost, get help immediately.

In the case of bright red and spurting blood loss, which is an indication that an artery has been cut, it is imperative for direct pressure to be applied to the wound, to elevate the injury as high as possible, and for the casualty to be taken directly to the hospital. If possible, ask the casualty to apply direct pressure to the wound so that you may assist in other ways. Definitely

"If there is uncontrollable bleeding with massive quantities of blood lost, get help immediately."

seek professional help; do not attempt to treat arterial bleeding solely on your own.

SEVERE PAIN

The severity of the pain does not always denote the severity of the injury, but it is often a good indicator. Either way, it is a modern comfort that pain can be controlled, for it can quickly become unbearable. Of course, it is not that long ago in human history that our only reliable method of pain control was the consumption of alcohol.

This method was far from optimal because in order to control severe pain, especially long-lasting pain, it was necessary to consume near deadly quantities of alcohol. This not only made the consumer quite ill, it also dramatically increased the time required for injuries to heal. Before the time when alcohol consumption became commonplace, there were very few remedies available for the control of pain, though every community had its own herbal medicines.

When there is a high degree of pain and the cause is not obvious, medical professionals can do the requisite testing to determine the problem. They have access to tools, laboratories, materials, experience, and team members that we simply do not. When the cause of the pain is known, it is the professionals who have the skills and the experience to rectify the situation.

Severe pain that is directly related to sports or exercise often is trauma related. Having the doctors treat the pain and the trauma injury at the same time only makes sense. If the pain is not accompanied by trauma, it is still a wise move to see the doctors in order to do adequate testing to determine the cause of the pain and to properly treat it.

Pain is a warning signal—a wakeup call from the body to let you know that something is not right. The louder the signal, the more urgently the body is attempting to get your attention in order to get you to correct the condition, force, substance, or influence that is resulting in pain. When pain is severe, it is often disabling, and can affect our ability to think clearly. Getting an objective outside viewpoint is often necessary to properly view the situation.

When all is said and done, there are extremely few instances, especially in the world of sports and exercise, where someone with severe pain should not be observed by a doctor. There is everything to gain and nothing to lose.

AVULSIONS

When there is a sudden, forceful stress placed on the skin, an "avulsion" can result. Essentially, this means that the skin, and often other tissue beneath the skin, literally "tore away" from itself. All but the most minor of avulsions usually require medical intervention.

BROKEN BONES

Accidents generally only take split seconds to occur. Assessing the damage usually takes far longer. Quite often, when a bone breaks, you have a sense of it, even if you aren't totally certain. Some bone breaks require virtually no first aid or remedial care other than the avoidance of pain. Some breaks definitely require medical attention. If you sustain an injury that you believe may be a broken bone, it is the smart thing to do to go directly to the doctor. In the case of many injuries, however, the fact that a bone was cracked is not immediately obvious.

Usually a broken bone is quite painful to touch at the location of the break. Functions related to the use of the bone may be impossible or extremely painful. There may be a visible lump under the skin indicating the location of the break and bone displacement. Hopefully, you will find no indications of broken bones.

Breaks: When to Get Help

Unlike arterial bleeding, where receiving medical attention is an absolute emergency, treating a broken bone can wait. Twelve to twenty-four hours is about the outside limit that one can delay in receiving care, however. The pain of a broken bone is not extremely great unless you "test" the function of that bone or stress the break in some fashion. The pain is also relatively long lasting, as the bone will not become stable for at least one to two weeks or longer.

If the break is not supported in a cast and you attempt to use the affected part during that time, it will be quite painful, or even impossible. If the break is properly supported in a cast so that it cannot be stressed, most of the pain will be gone in three to five days.

Most people go directly to the doctor if they even suspect a broken bone. This is probably a wise decision, but there is a bit of wiggle room available for people who just hate going to the doctor for "unnecessary" care. There are certain bone breaks for which the doctors typically offer very little or no care whatever. The following fractures often need and receive little care at the doctor that cannot be provided at home:

Rib Fractures

Ribs are long, U-shaped, and rather delicate bones. If pressured or bumped in too severe a fashion, they display a propensity for cracking near their midpoint. The middle of the rib is at your side, about where your arm touches when it is hanging freely. A fractured rib will be tender to touch at the precise location of the break. It will also feel tender at the broken spot when the rib is compressed from its two ends simultaneously, at the front and at the back. Breathing is painful when a rib is fractured, as this causes the broken bone ends to be put into motion.

Ribs also fracture towards their very front end, at or near the point where they attach to the sternum via cartilage. The care for this type of fracture is similar to that of a rib that is fractured at its midpoint.

Broken ribs cannot be placed in a cast. Being wrapped with an elastic bandage can provide support for them. This can easily be done at home. Be prepared to reposition or remove the wrap should it become uncomfortable. Because rib fractures are constantly in motion due to breathing, they are generally slower to heal than most broken bones and can be more painful. Expect six to eight weeks of ever-diminishing discomfort from a fractured rib before it is fully healed.

It should be stressed that most rib fractures are simple and require little attention. However, some can be very dangerous or even life threatening. *Do not attempt to treat any of the following rib fractures.* Go for immediate medical assistance or help the victim get to the hospital as quickly as possible in the event of:

Multiple Rib Fractures

When more than one and definitely more than two ribs are broken, the rib cage is in danger of losing its stability.

Displaced Fracture

If there is an obvious bump, deformity, or displacement of bone under the skin. If the broken rib breaks through the skin, this open fracture will result in a sucking wound.

Sucking Wound

Named for sound of air being sucked into the chest that often accompanies a penetrating chest wound. Rib fractures and/or a collapsed lung, may or may not, accompany this condition.

Crushed Chest

This condition can come about as a result of multiple rib fractures.

Paroxysmal Breathing

Also resulting from multiple rib fractures, this condition is seen when the rib cage goes in while the victim breathes in, and out when the victim breathes out, the opposite pattern of normal breathing.

Asphyxia

In the case of a broken rib, the development of asphyxia, a deficiency of oxygen in the body, could indicate a collapsed lung or damage to a vital organ.

Shock

Experiencing mild shock after any injury, and certainly following the fracture of a bone, is completely normal. Shock is indicated by the appearance of: paleness, cold moist skin, weakness or a giddy feeling, weak rapid pulse, shallow breathing, and yawning. Should the degree of shock become severe, especially to the point of the casualty vomiting or losing consciousness, seek immediate medical attention.

METATARSAL AND TARSAL FRACTURES

Each foot has five tarsal bones (one leading to each toe) and each toe has three (metatarsal) bones. These quite thin and small bones fracture relatively easily. From the littlest toe to the largest (fifth to first), the bones get progressively thicker and stronger. Most of the force of walking and running is transferred across the largest of these bones. If the third, fourth or fifth metatarsal bone breaks, and there is no displacement of bone, some people find that they are fine to abstain from medical treatment.

Other people prefer the safety and security of having the foot placed in a cast. If no care is taken, a few days of bed rest with the foot elevated and wrapped is recommended. After that, keeping the foot taped or wrapped for about three weeks helpful. During that time, moving carefully, limping slightly or using a cane, and avoiding all painful movements will suffice. As long as the fracture is not open and there is no obvious displacement of bone, it is possible to avoid seeking medical attention for breaks to any of the metatarsal bones.

It must be stressed again that obtaining professional medical assistance for any wound or injury is always prudent. Not getting medical advice should always be considered the riskier option.

TYPES OF BREAKS AND FRACTURES

The term "fracture," when referring to bone, can mean either a cracked or broken bone. Fractures may be caused by direct or indirect force. A direct fracture is one that occurs exactly where the force is applied to the bone, such as what happens when a rock falls on your foot.

An indirect fracture can occur in three ways: some distance from the point of impact, as in breaking your arm when falling on your hands; when a muscle pulls violently on a bone, as in breaking the kneecap by accidently kicking the ground instead of a ball; and when twisting or rotating force causes a bone to break, as may accompany a sprained ankle.

There are essentially only two types of fractures, open and closed. With an open fracture, bones are exposed to the outside environment due to a break in the skin. The skin remains intact in the case of a closed fracture.

The amount of damage done by the break is not dependent upon whether the break is open or closed. Blood vessels, nerves, organs and other vital structures can be severely damaged by sharp broken bones in a closed fracture.

It's a good idea to familiarize yourself with a book on first aid, which will describe the exact care procedures for dealing with fractures of the various bones of the body. Essentially, the idea is to immobilize, support, and sufficiently pad the area, so that the patient can be transported to get professional help painlessly, and with minimal risk of additional injury.

Greenstick Fractures

Bones break very much like the branches of a tree. The older branches are more prone to breaking, as are older bones. Young branches, such as those on a sapling tree, will bend and even twist quite a lot before breaking.

A young person's bones are still quite malleable in this way too. Their bones will bend and "give" to forces that might break the bones of their grandparents. One type of break that is uncommon in adults and not as unusual in children is called a "greenstick" fracture. Usually the result of twisting force (hence, sometimes an alert signal to possible child abuse), the greenstick fracture is unusual because like its namesake, the bone breaks into many long spiral-shaped pieces, much as a sapling branch would split apart if twisted.

Displaced Breaks

When bones break, the ends either stay in place and in alignment with each other or they don't. It is much simpler when the bones remain aligned, of course, and the amount of care required by the physician is then reduced dramatically. However, if the bones are displaced, even a little bit, it is a good idea to have them "set" by a physician. It is not absolutely essential, as the bones will likely heal to each other and eventually straighten out suitably even if they are not set, but the entire process runs much smoother and faster when the ends are replaced. The doctor cannot do the actual healing, only your body can do that.

There are special cells that rebuild the bone, known as osteoblasts. The osteoclasts break down bone. These two specific types of cells actually take bone away from where it is not needed and replace it where it is needed in order to "straighten" out a displaced break that healed improperly. Replacing the two bone ends is a better arrangement, however, because it allows the bone to resume its original length, whereas otherwise the displaced ends of a broken bone could overlap each other by an inch or more.

Partial Breaks

Most of the breaks that occur in bones are partial breaks, rather than complete ones. These small fractures are still quite uncomfortable for a few weeks after they occur. The bone does not end up in two pieces, but a visible crack can be seen on an X-ray. A bone with a partial break is delicate and it should be treated that way for three to four weeks; the fracture can easily become complete if it is stressed too much.

Shatters

Though rare, it's possible for bone to shatter like glass. I know of one person whose tibia (in her lower leg) shattered into about two hundred pieces when she lost her balance stepping off of a four-inch step. As mentioned earlier, covering every possible injury is not the primary concern of this book. For that, a book on first aid would be more appropriate. For the purposes of this book, it is important to understand two things about broken bone injuries.

When bones break, they should be supported, protected, and cleaned if necessary, and the victim taken to a doctor for professional care. A broken bone is likely to take three to six weeks or longer to heal, depending upon the nature of the break, the vitality of the individual, and the degree of rest and proper recovery conditions that are supplied. The break is extremely vulnerable to reinjury for the first two weeks after it initially occurs.

Newly Broken Bones

Newly broken bones should not be stressed or irritated in any way.

Even mild vibrations will prove extremely painful, as the nerves around the bone in the area of the break become extremely sensitive. When bony material is laid down in and around the break, it is initially similar to wet cement, or ketchup. Like any colloid, if it is vibrated, shaken, or stressed in any way, the solid and liquid matter will separate and what was once soft, but semi-solid, will turn into a liquid. Healing is impeded every time this happens to a broken bone. This is why splinting and casting bones encourages speedy healing.

Bones heal in much the same way that the skin does. A scab must form, stabilizing the break, and then new bone material can be placed into the bone in order to connect one end of the break to the other. The scab, when it forms around the outside of the bone, is referred to as a callus. The callus begins to form almost immediately after the bone breaks, but takes about two weeks to form completely. On an X-ray, the callus becomes visible after about a week, a sure sign that a bone was broken or that bone integrity was interrupted. The callus will remain on the bone for a lifetime, like a scar. It will be another two to four weeks before the bone is fully healed, in general.

Until the callus is fully formed and there is no more pain upon use, it is wise to limit or avoid stressing a healing bone. It's better to wait an extra few days than to suffer a re-break of an already broken bone. Caution must be taken during all activities not to hurt the break, even inadvertently. While movement and activities must remain limited during the time a bone is healing, it does not mean that training need be reduced.

A broken arm will not slow you down for running, at least not after the first few days. A broken leg provides a wonderful opportunity to do upper body strength training and even some lower body flexibility training. Rather than seeing them as an excuse to become inactive, try to envision the training opportunity that every injury brings you.

HEAD INJURY

Concussion and Loss of Consciousness

Nothing will catch your attention more than a hard hit on the head. A solid blow to the body can also be considered to have concussive force, and can do considerable damage, both internal and external. But it is hits to the head that give us the most concern. The bones of the skull are fairly strong, especially at the back and front, which is where they are most likely to get hit. The skin may break and there might be a lot of bleeding in the case of almost any head injury, but these are not our major concern. Concussion to the brain is where the potential for serious damage lies.

The brain is a colloid, meaning that it is a solid material that will turn to a liquid if subjected to severe shaking or a powerful concussive force. The brain and spinal cord, which make up the central nervous system, are so important to the functioning of the body that they are the only organs that are completely encased inside a bony "shell." To keep the brain even more protected and insulated from bumps and bruises, there is a layer of liquid between the brain and the skull known as cerebrospinal fluid that stabilizes the brain within the skull.

When we experience a hard hit to the skull, however, it is possible for the brain to actually bump against the inside of the skull. This bumping of the brain against the skull results in the injury we refer to as concussion.

Concussion, sometimes referred to as "brain shaking," usually results from a blow to the head or jaw, or from a hard fall, often from a height. Usually concussion is accompanied by at least momentary unconsciousness, but it can be of such short duration that the trauma victim has no memory of going unconscious at all.

If you see someone take a hard hit to the head or jaw, or fall hard and bang his or her head, a thorough check for concussion is warranted. The injured party should be observed closely for a substantial period of time. Should any of the signs or symptoms of concussion be displayed, take the casualty to the doctor immediately.

Signs and symptoms of concussion include a brief or partial loss of consciousness. While the casualty is unconscious, watch for the following signs: shallow breathing, paleness, cold or clammy skin, and a weak or rapid pulse. Once consciousness is regained, the casualty may experience nausea or vomiting. Ask for memory-related details of the injury. If the casualty cannot remember the events immediately before or after the injury, or doesn't know the answers to questions about the date, time, or present location, suspect concussion.

If a person seems to be recovering well from a concussion, place him/her in the care of a responsible person. Advise the casualty to see a doctor. If recovery is not as rapid as would be hoped, take the casualty directly to the hospital. Compression injuries of the brain or fractures of the skull are distinct possibilities.

The amount of damage incurred from a concussion depends greatly upon which part of the brain hits the skull, and how hard it hits. Loss of consciousness is a fair indicator of degree of damage. Most doctors agree that there is a direct proportional relationship between the length of time spent unconscious and the amount of damage done in a concussion. Take anyone to the hospital if they go unconscious from a concussion.

If they are only unconscious for a few seconds and refuse to go to the hospital when they come to, they should be watched closely for any unusual behavior. Sleepiness, visual disturbances, unclear or slurred speech, lack of coordination, or anything else that leaves the observer wary, warrants a trip to the hospital. There could be swelling on the brain, internal bleeding inside the cranium, or any number of other very serious complications from a concussion. Do not hesitate to be overly cautious when it comes to head injuries; chances are you will never regret it.

Other than concussion, there are two primary head injuries that we must be on the lookout for in the world of sports and exercise injuries. These are compression injuries and skull fractures.

Compression Injury

A compression injury to the brain is a very serious condition which develops when pressure is exerted on the brain. It is possible to have brain compression as a result of a skull fracture, which is called a depressed fracture, where a piece of bone is actually pressing upon the brain, but this is the least common option. More commonly there is bleeding inside the cranium or the brain itself swells. Any of these three possibilities could follow after a concussion, but concussion is not a requirement for compression on the brain. Brain compression can take hours and even days to develop after any head injury.

Symptoms of brain compression include: a deteriorating level of responsiveness, possible noisy breathing, full but slow pulse, unequal pupil size and responsiveness, one-sided weakness or paralysis, a flushed but dry face, and a rise in temperature. If someone you know has taken a hard blow to the head and is experiencing any or all of the above-mentioned symptoms, take him or her to the hospital immediately.

Skull Fracture

A skull fracture is a severe enough injury that there will likely be many other repercussions, including possible concussion, brain compression, and contusion (bruising) of the brain. Blood or cerebrospinal fluid may leak from the person's nose or ears, or blood may stain the whites of the eyes.

A person with a skull fracture usually requires a definitive diagnosis via X-ray, but will generally demonstrate the symptoms of the problems mentioned above. In addition, a soft "boggy" zone or a depression of the scalp in the area of the fracture may be discovered upon gentle palpation of the wound. Anyone with a suspected skull fracture should be taken immediately to the hospital.

POTENTIAL FOR INTERNAL INJURY

With every blow to the body or head, there is potential for serious internal injuries. Usually there are reliable signs and symptoms that give indications that something is wrong. Being familiar with those symptoms and signs, and knowing how to interpret them, is an important part of being in the responsible position of caring for another human being.

Visceral Injury

While this type of injury is not a common one to exercise or sports injuries, it certainly is possible, and severe enough that it deserves mention. A hard hit to the chest, kidneys, or to the upper or lower abdomen, can result in serious damage to the organs local to that area. Complaints of pain, nausea, vomiting, unexpected blood loss, or signs of shock, should be considered serious for anyone who has experienced a hard blow to the chest, abdomen, or kidney area. Demonstration of such symptoms is cause for alarm. These persons should be transported immediately to the hospital.

Internal Bleeding

Internal bleeding of organs such as the kidneys, liver, or spleen can follow a hard hit to the body that leaves no trace of external evidence. Internal bleeding can be just as serious, and sometimes more serious, than external bleeding. The accumulating blood is lost to the circulatory system while it can be putting pressure upon the brain or preventing proper function of the lungs, or even the heart.

After any violent hit, always be aware of the possibility of internal bleeding. Though no blood may be visible, sometimes the accumulation of blood is discernable or palpable around the area where contact was made. Suspect internal bleeding if any signs or symptoms of shock are displayed after any sports-related collision. Transport the victim to the hospital as rapidly as possible.

"IN-BETWEEN" INJURIES

Every time we incur an injury, no matter if it is big or small, we must note it, assess it, and determine the type of care, if any, that it requires. Most injuries are easy to deal with: they either require little to no care or they need to be dealt with by professionals.

Little thought is required in deciding to clean and apply an adhesive bandage to a scrape or in deciding to take someone with gaping wounds, heavy bleeding, bones broken through the skin, or other such injuries, directly to the hospital. Injuries that fall in the middle of these parameters can give us trouble, for when we are presented with these "in-between" injuries, there are important and sometimes difficult decisions to be made. Such in-between situations can be sticky, and it is those that we address now.

"Every time we incur an injury, no matter if it is big or small, we must note it, assess it, and determine the type of care, if any, that it requires."

An injury improperly dealt with can leave a lifetime of repercussions. Following are several examples of accidents and how they were handled.

- I was walking alongside the road in my hometown one day when I saw a teenage boy weave into traffic on his bicycle. He got hit head-on and flew about 15 or more feet into the air, landing on his knees on the asphalt and then hitting his back and head before finally bouncing onto the grass. I was the first one on the scene. One look at him and I knew the damage was serious, though incredibly he was not hurt as badly as I had imagined he would be. There was no skin on his knees, but except for being dazed, he appeared otherwise unharmed. I told him I was there to help, and to "just sit where you are" while another passerby phoned for help. He was conscious, not bleeding, and nothing appeared broken. Within two minutes, paramedics were on the scene. The hospital cleaned and dressed his abrasions, and released him later that same day.
- I was bicycling with a friend down a long, steep hill on a quiet road when his front rim gave way. He tumbled head over heels repeatedly on the asphalt. By the time I'd stopped my bike and gotten back up the hill to him, he was holding his hand on his chin. I checked him everywhere and all I found were abrasions—lots of them. Road rash is uncomfortable, but not usually serious. When he took his hand off of his chin I saw it was split wide open but had not yet begun to bleed. I took a folded neckerchief and had him hold it on his chin, applying pressure. I stood in the road and stopped the next car that passed and asked the driver to take my friend to the nearest hospital, which he did. I followed by bicycle. After a thorough cleansing of the road rash and eighty-something stitches in his chin later, he was released.

- A friend of mine fell on her head at a party. She did not lose consciousness even for a moment. She seemed really dazed and appeared to be going into shock. Her pulse was racing and thready, her pupils were unresponsive to a penlight, and she was suddenly very sleepy. We took her to the hospital. Hospitals being what they are, service was extremely slow. After an hour, we finally got a room, but after another two hours, still she had not been seen by a doctor. My friend was quite animated by now, and seemed to have totally recovered her senses. After four hours she finally said, "let's go," so we left the hospital and took her home. The next day and thereafter she was completely fine.
- During the warm-ups of a gymnastics competition, one of the competitors fell from the horizontal bar and landed on his back and head, on the mats. He blacked out and remained unconscious for what seemed a long time but was probably only about 20 seconds. He was unhurt in any other way and when he came to he seemed perfectly fine. He opted to stay with his team for the duration of the meet, but did not compete. He did not seek subsequent medical care and was fine thereafter.
- I was in Israel on vacation. On the beach one day, I walked out to a huge breakwater built of rocks via a connecting sandbar. It seemed perfectly safe until an exceptionally big wave washed right over me. In the resultant fall, a rock punctured my shin, making a fairly deep hole about the size of a finger. I went to my hotel room, washed up, and lay down on the floor with my calf resting on my bed. The bleeding stopped completely as long as I stayed lying down. Each time I stood, the bleeding started again. I was in no rush to go to the hospital, and not in much pain. It took almost twelve hours for the bleeding to stop. The next day, when I went walking, I kept the puncture covered and wrapped. Of Price's rules, I used: pressure, rest, elevation, and support, to my advantage.

Note that bleeding sometimes takes longer to stop than you would like it to. Of course, the amount of blood being lost is crucial. Minor bleeding that won't stop, as is typical of a cut from a very sharp surface, is usually nothing more than a nuisance. Once again, it is the "in-between" situation that requires intelligent thought and action.

Knowing that an injury has been properly cared for is just as important as the quality of the actual care. Confidence can be sensed, like a dog can sense fear, and when the caregiver is confident, so is the patient. If you are the person on whom the first-aid responsibilities often fall, it is to your advantage to take a first-aid course. Feel free to blend the guidelines given in that course with the information offered in this chapter, and to mix both with substantial portions of common sense.

There are truly no generic guidelines for seeking professional help that apply in every situation. Each injury is unique, as is each person. Decisions about getting help must be based upon those unique circumstances. Still, prudent caution is always a smart move. No one looks stupid for asking for help, even if it turns out that none is needed. If, on the other hand, one does not seek medical attention when it would have been useful, looking stupid may end up being the least of your concerns.

12. Weather-Induced Injury Propensities

Just when you have sorted out your training gear and perfected your masterpiece training routine, the weather pops in and introduces more variables. In most places on the planet, "if you don't like the weather, wait a few minutes," applies, but it could not be truer than it is in the United Kingdom, where I live for much of the year. I have learned that if you are not prepared for the weather, it can seriously hurt you.

I recently went out for a run on a beautiful and warm autumn afternoon. It had rained all morning and when it stopped, there was a blue sky, an encouragingly peaceful rainbow, and calm weather. After I had been running for only a few minutes, clouds blew in on a fresh, strong wind. Shortly thereafter, it started raining, almost horizontally, and the temperature dropped quickly.

I turned and headed home. Before I could get there, large hailstones were pummeling me mercilessly and I was slipping and sliding on the pavement. I arrived home in the midst of a torrential downpour. By the time I had showered, it was beautiful and calm out again. When I went for a walk later in the day, it had turned into a warm, sunny afternoon.

The following information and considerations cover a great many of the weather possibilities for which you must be prepared, but certainly not all of them.

You'll note that dehydration is an issue in most of the weather conditions mentioned below. Rather than repeat the information presented on dehydration in Chapters 6 and 8, only a short mention of dehydration is made in the relevant categories; however, the different physiological demands created by each weather or atmospheric condition are noted. Hopefully, this information will together show how any instance of dehydration represents a serious concern.

HEAT: DEHYDRATION, EXHAUSTION, AND STROKE

Although heat is more of an issue in tropical and subtropical zones, it can affect you almost anywhere you live, at least at certain times of the year. The two main health concerns that are caused by heat—heat exhaustion and heat stroke—begin with dehydration.

Heat exhaustion is serious enough, but heat stroke will quickly put an end to your day's activities, and will likely have an adverse impact upon you for several days to come. It is best to avoid heat exhaustion and heat stroke entirely by recognizing their early warning symptoms and completely relieving them before they get started.

RECOGNIZING SYMPTOMS

The basic symptoms of heat exhaustion and heat stroke are similar: exhaustion accompanied by restlessness, headache, dizziness, and nausea. Where they differ is that with heat exhaustion, which is usually caused by a loss of minerals and water from the body, there is usually paleness, cramps, cold or clammy skin, and a rapid, weak pulse. Body temperature in heat exhaustion may be no higher than normal, or can even be cool. Fainting is not uncommon in severe heat exhaustion.

A heat stroke victim will have many of the same symptoms as

someone with heat exhaustion. Symptoms will differ in that the victim will usually complain of feeling hot, have dry lips and dry skin, have very high body temperature (above 104°F, with up to 109°F and beyond possible), have a bounding pulse, and possibly have noisy breathing. The heat stroke victim is likely to develop unconsciousness suddenly and it can be very deep. Heat stroke is the result of the body no longer being able to cool itself via normal means. We often see this occurring in environments with high temperature, high humidity, and low air circulation.

PREVENTION AND CARE

Prevention is the name of the game when it comes to heat-related issues. Wetting the head, hair, and even the entire body, helps to pull off excess heat. In extremely sunny conditions, wearing a hat and light clothing, and keeping it wet, will also help keep you cool. The consumption of sufficient water and mineral-rich foods, such as fruits and vegetables, is essential. We can lose as much as a gallon of water in one to two hours of heavy exertion. The loss of half a gallon is sufficient to set off heat exhaustion or heat stroke in some people. If you are going to be active in extremely hot weather, drink water before your exertions begin and throughout the period of activity.

Pour or sponge water onto your head and body as you go, or wet your head under a hose or spigot. Replace lost water weight immediately upon finishing your activity by drinking water again. Remember that heat exhaustion results from a loss of minerals as well as water. Celery is an excellent vegetable for replacing sodium, and bananas are excellent for replacing potassium. The two foods, blended together with water, make the best electrolyte replacement fluid.

Should you see someone fall victim to heat exhaustion, lay the person down, preferably in the shade. Offer sips of cool water. They should not drink rapidly, but continue to drink until rehydrated. If celery is available, offer it, as even a few bites will help. If celery is not an option, a few grains of straight table salt may help replace the missing sodium, although there are mixed thoughts on this as it may also cause dehydration. In all instances, keep the victim completely resting.

A person who falls ill to heat stroke should also be put into a cool place, preferably where there is shade and wind, or moving air. Clothing should be wetted or removed until the body temperature drops to 100°F or less.

In heat exhaustion and heat stroke, the casualty should be offered professional medical assistance once immediate first-aid measures are taken.

COLD: HYPOTHERMIA AND FROSTBITE

Exposure to environmental cold can be just as debilitating, and often leaves a more permanent impairment, than exposure to heat. Damage from cold is easily prevented. All it takes is some forethought. The symptoms of hypothermia tend to come on rather gradually, so one must be diligent in keeping a lookout for them. While damage from cold exposure is typically most severe on a wintry mountainside or in open areas, it can just as easily occur anywhere on a cold winter's day or night.

RECOGNIZING SYMPTOMS

Because the symptoms of hypothermia accrue gradually, and are often subtle, one must be vigilant when watching for them. Shivering is one of the earliest signs, and is usually followed by pale, cold, and dry skin. By definition, hypothermia occurs when the body temperature drops 2°F or more. As pulse and respiration rates slow, the victim may exhibit odd or irrational behavior. Eventually, unconsciousness ensues and is followed by cessation of breathing and stoppage of the heart.

Frostbite usually occurs in the extremities or to exposed areas of the body that have limited circulation, such as fingers, toes, the tips of the ears, and the nose. These parts will first turn pale, then waxy white, and later turn blue. They will eventually go black if left untreated. Blisters may occur. The victim will usually complain of "pins and needles" or intense pain that will gradually diminish as the affected parts go numb with cold. The frostbitten areas will eventually become hard to the touch as they literally freeze solid.

PREVENTION AND CARE

Hypothermia and frostbite are quite easy to prevent. Accordingly, there should rarely be a need to care for these conditions. Hypothermia is basically a case of a drop in core temperature. Using multiple layers of clothing can prevent this. The innermost layers should be "breathable" and preferably allow "wicking" to prevent perspiration from accumulating.

"Hypothermia and frostbite are quite easy to prevent."

Another method of allowing excess moisture to escape is by wearing a loose-fitting neck and sleeved top. Some high-tech gear will also have vents under the arms for this purpose. Keeping the body warm is of primary importance, so extra layers on the torso are most effective. Dry socks, a hat, and gloves, all help prevent heat loss, thus sparing heat for the torso. In extremely cold weather, it is better to err on the side of being too warm than being too cold. You can always remove an excess layer or open a coat to cool off if necessary. Generating heat through physical exertion will help stave off hypothermia.

As mentioned earlier, frostbite generally affects the extremities. Even if the torso is warm, frostbite can affect the fingers, toes, ears, or nose. Protect these areas as best as possible by covering them with clothing and not exposing them to the wind. In situations of extreme cold, go indoors frequently and warm yourself thoroughly. Change to dry socks and dry gloves as needed.

Treatment for hypothermia involves raising core temperature. Take the person indoors, if possible. Change their clothing, if at all moist, to dry, warm, and loose-fitting ones. Use a hot-water bottle, and place it on the left side of the body, under the arm, or on the sternum to best warm core circulation. A warm bath will bring about a more rapid rise in body temperature, but take care that it not be excessively hot. The consumption of a warm drink such as tea, warm juice, or even warm water will help. Do not heat fingers or toes, as this will increase blood flow to the limbs, and may result in a drop in core temperature.

Frostbite must be treated in its early stages or it becomes very serious business. In the early stages, simply warm the affected part. If it is a finger or hand, put the hand under the opposite arm until normal color and feeling returns. For other areas, warm them by going indoors, by giving them better protective covering, or by putting on a warm compress of some type.

Warm compresses can be made from any hot liquid in a zipper-type bag, a warm rock wrapped in cloth, or by using the chemical hand warmers that are commercially available. Putting the affected part under warm running water works well in the earliest stages of frostbite. The treatment of the advanced stages of frostbite is beyond the scope of this book.

ALTITUDE: OXYGEN DEPRIVATION AND DEHYDRATION

As you head upward in altitude, the concentration of the air molecules becomes thinner. The percentage of oxygen relative to everything else that is in air remains the same, there is just less air overall. The air becomes increasingly thin until at some point, around 15,000 feet above sea level for most people, it becomes difficult to function without breathing in additional oxygen. People who are "acclimated" to the altitude can likely function at a few thousand feet higher.

Thin air is not always easy to perceive. It's somewhat easier to inhale and exhale because it's thinner, but for most people this is not noticeable. Basically, it feels just like any other air except that you get out of breath exceptionally easily. At ten thousand feet, simple tasks

"At ten thousand feet, simple tasks such as walking up a flight of stairs or bending over to tie your shoe, are often enough to leave you winded."

such as walking up a flight of stairs or bending over to tie your shoe, are often enough to leave you winded.

At altitude, the humidity tends to stay fairly low. Water evaporates more rapidly so we lose it without noticing the loss. Breathing at altitude requires extra water from our system to keep the airways moisturized. More water is lost with each exhale in the high and dry climates usually found between five thousand and ten thousand feet than is lost at sea level. Dehydration can quickly become a serious issue at altitude. You may wish to reread Chapters 6 and 8 for relevant discussions about dehydration.

Dehydration compounds the challenge of getting sufficient oxygen to your cells because the blood volume is reduced, resulting in thicker blood that is less efficient at flowing through the capillaries. At altitude, where reduced oxygen supply is the major problem, dehydration becomes an important concern. The consumption of salty foods, dehydrated foods, alcohol, or any other dehydrating influences, should be curtailed if you are a visitor to a high-altitude environment. Becoming fully acclimated to living in high-altitude environments can take four to six months. Until that much time has passed, it is better to err on the side of caution regarding staying hydrated when you are at altitude.

Oxygen deprivation to the cells is the main concern at altitude, and like hydration issues, this problem becomes progressively more severe the higher in altitude you go. The condition where there is not enough oxygen getting to the cells of the body is referred to as "asphyxia." As mentioned in Chapter 8, the ability of the blood to uptake, transport, and deliver oxygen to the cells goes down as the amount of fat in the blood goes up. If you are visiting a high-altitude area, eating fatty foods is not in your best interest.

RECOGNIZING SYMPTOMS

Asphyxia due to visiting a high elevation is referred to as "altitude sickness." Symptoms vary, but the primary one is an unrelenting headache. This may be accompanied by extreme tiredness, loss of appetite, nausea, weakness, an inability to catch one's breath, thirst, and in severe instances, blueness around the lips and fingertips.

PREVENTION AND CARE

The body adapts to altitude by increasing the number of red blood cells. This happens most efficiently during the recovery phases of our day, when we are at rest or asleep. If you know you are going to visit a location that is extremely high in altitude, it is a good idea to be well-rested when you do so, and to get plenty of sleep while you are there. Also, be sure to remain well-hydrated before, during, and after your visit.

The omission of overtly fatty foods from your diet for 48 hours before going to altitude will make a noticeable difference in how well you handle the altitude, as it often takes that long for dietary fat to reach, and be cleared from, the bloodstream. Eating a relatively low-fat diet while you are at altitude will also be of assistance in keeping altitude sickness at bay. The consumption of alcoholic beverages, salty foods, or other dehydrating factors is also contraindicated. By keeping your oxygen demands minimal for the first day or two of a high-altitude visit, you give your body the maximum chance at adapting.

Exercising aggressively when you first get to your high-altitude location is therefore not recommended. Once you do start exercising, increase the demands you place upon your system gradually, making sure that you fully recover each night.

If altitude sickness does overcome you, there are a few options. You can go to bed and try to sleep it off, being sure to stay well-hydrated and following all the other lifestyle suggestions. Sometimes, breathing bottled oxygen for a few minutes will help. This can be done several times per day, if needed, until all symptoms subside. The only other solution is to go to a location that has a lower altitude, preferably one that is at five thousand feet or lower. In extreme cases, a helicopter airlift may be required.

SUN: BURN, GLARE DAMAGE, AND DEHYDRATION

As with most environmental and weather factors, exposure to the sun greatly increases your need for water and multiplies your risk of dehydration. The sun is a powerfully drying force, and should not be underestimated. The physiological adaptations made by the body in response to exposure to sunlight also require that additional water be consumed. Refer to Chapters 6 and 8 for details on managing your water needs.

Glare from the sun can cause painful damage to the cornea of the eye and even temporary blindness. Although typically referred to as "snow blindness," this condition can have many other causes. In environments where the sunlight can be reflected—on light-colored sand, near water, from the road, on the hood of a vehicle or hull of a boat, off of white rocks, from the glass of buildings or vehicles, or perhaps most intensely, from snow and ice—the glare can be multiplied immensely. Snow blindness will be the result, even if it happens in a hot desert.

In many warm locations that function as tourist destinations, the most common reason for people to visit the hospital is because of sunburn. Sunburn can range from mildly uncomfortable to seriously debilitating. I met one man in Key West, Florida, who had been sunburned so badly that he had to spend three weeks in the hospital recovering. He had even been living in Key West for six months prior to getting burned, and thought he had acquired a very good tan. On the night before his burn, he had gone to a beach party and fallen asleep on the sand. When he awoke the next afternoon, he went straight to the hospital.

The sun emits several different types of ultraviolet rays. Some elicit a tanning response while others simply burn the skin. It's important to understand when and where these rays are most prevalent in order to reduce the likelihood of sunburn. Cumulatively, sunburn can pose more than just a minor inconvenience; it can cause serious damage to the skin, and possibly result in irreversible skin conditions. While melanoma and the other most serious skin cancers have been repeatedly shown to be prevented by sun exposure, certain other types of skin cancers may have their roots in repeated bouts of sunburn.

"Sunburn can range from mildly uncomfortable to seriously debilitating."

RECOGNIZING SYMPTOMS

The symptoms of sunburn develop incrementally. Be alert for sunburn as the spring weather starts to heat up. The lower angle of the sun in spring and autumn actually allows more burning rays to penetrate the atmosphere than when the sun is closer to straight above, as it is in summer. One of the first signs of sunburn is that the skin begins to turn red, and it may also become blotchy due to dilation of the capillary beds. Eventually, sunburned skin will become hot, itchy, swollen, tender, and may even blister. A casualty of sunburn may feel hot or feverish, and will be extremely sensitive to the sun for several days following being burned.

A victim of snow blindness will complain of pain in the eyes and sometimes a gritty feeling in the eyes. The eyes will likely be red, watering, and very sensitive to light. If asked, someone with snow blindness will almost always mention recent exposure to an inordinate amount of glare.

PREVENTION AND CARE

The easiest prevention for sunburn is to avoid getting more sun than your skin is ready to handle. The judicious use of a hat, umbrella, and protective clothing can completely obviate the need for any chemical sunblock creams or lotions. If you have a spot that is particularly prone to sunburn, such as your nose, plain zinc ointment will effectively stop the sun's rays. Take advantage of the shade, as needed. A good rule of thumb that if your shadow is longer than your height, the sun is relatively safe for you, unless you have extremely sensitive skin. One of the healthiest ways to avoid sunburn is to maintain at least a light tan year-round.

Should you become sunburned, proceed to the shade as soon as possible. Cool the skin with the application of a wet cloth, or by taking a cool shower. If the burned skin requires treatment, the application of aloe vera or a similar burn cream is appropriate. Be sure to drink sips of cool water and to make sure that you are not overheated. Most important is to stay out of the sun until the burn is completely healed. If the skin continues to blister repeatedly or the sunburn pain is more than can be tolerated, seek medical attention.

The use of a broad-brimmed hat plus sunglasses, ski goggles, mountaineering glasses, or even specifically designed glare goggles, is the best method for preventing snow blindness. The object is to limit the amount of light that actually reaches the eyes. Mountaineering glasses have ultra dark-lenses and usually have blinders on the sides to reduce the total amount of light that reaches the eyes. Glare goggles have opaque lenses with very small slit openings through which only limited amounts of light can enter.

Should you experience snow blindness, the first thing to do is to go to a place where the light is minimized. Then simply bathe the eyes in cool water and keep the eyes closed for a while. The application of eye pads or any cloth to keep out light is useful. If the eyes do not recover within several hours, seek medical attention.

HUMIDITY: PROSTRATION AND DEHYDRATION

When exercising in conditions of high heat and relatively high humidity, perspiration may not evaporate as quickly as is forms. In this case, the perspiration will drip rather than evaporate, and thus not perform its cooling function as well. Quite often, this will lead to greater quantities of perspiration forming, and subsequently dripping off of the body. A substantial quantity of water and sodium can be lost relatively rapidly in this fashion. Whenever there are significant water losses, dehydration must be considered as a very real possibility. Heat exhaustion, which also can be referred to as heat prostration, comes about due to the heavy losses of water and sodium that are the main ingredients in sweat.

"Heat exhaustion, which also can be referred to as heat prostration, comes about due to the heavy losses of water and sodium that are the main ingredients in sweat."

RECOGNIZING SYMPTOMS

See Chapters 6 and 8 for further information on dehydration. The symptoms of heat prostration are the same as those given earlier in this chapter for heat exhaustion and heat stroke.

PREVENTION AND CARE

Prevention of dehydration in situations of extreme heat and high humidity includes those guidelines already given plus the additional consumption of a sodium source. Celery is one of the richest and most healthful sources of sodium. A drink of celery juice blended with water makes a very good electrolyte replacement fluid.

To prevent heat exhaustion under conditions of high humidity, take advantage of other methods of keeping the body cool. If a windy spot is available for exercise, it is preferable to a spot that is in the lee of the wind. Exercise in the shade if possible, or wear a wide-brimmed hat. Take frequent cool showers, or exercise in the water if it is available. Drink cool or cold drinks if they are available, and wet your head and clothing repeatedly. Be sure to be fully hydrated and well-nourished with minerals before starting to exercise in the heat and humidity. Exercise early in the day, or in the evening, rather than at midday whenever possible.

Care of heat prostration and dehydration were given earlier in this chapter.

WIND: BURN AND MORE DEHYDRATION

Windburn is uncomfortable, but rarely is it dangerous. The wind can be very dehydrating to exposed areas, even to the point of damaging the skin. Coupled with damage from the sun, windburn can prove extremely uncomfortable. The lips are especially vulnerable to windburn, and will tend to crack and become chapped from extended exposure unless they are protected.

The wind can be exceptionally dehydrating. When the weather is dry, whether in cold conditions or in hot, the wind can be even more of a dehydrating factor.

RECOGNIZING SYMPTOMS

See Chapters 6 and 8 for more details of the signs and symptoms of dehydration.

Dry lips, chapped lips, burning cheeks, and any dry, exposed skin could be symptoms of windburn, but are not necessarily so. As there are many other factors that can result in the same or similar symptoms, the primary warning for windburn is extended exposure to high and/or dry winds.

PREVENTION AND CARE

For prevention and care of wind-related or other forms of dehydration, see the relevant portions of Chapters 6 and 8. For prevention of windburn, minimize wind exposure for sensitive parts such as the eyes, ears, face, and especially the lips by covering them with protective clothing or creams. There are excellent lip and skin glosses that will provide combined protection from both the wind and the sun, if desired.

The areas that are most likely to be damaged by the wind are also areas that heal exceptionally rapidly, as a rule. Remove the cause of the problem and the body will heal itself, in most cases. Ointment or creams can be used to sooth any skin that was chapped or cracked by wind.

UNDERWATER AND OTHER BAROMETRIC CONSIDERATIONS

There are unique problems posed when exercising underwater and at extremely high altitudes. Nitrogen narcosis and asphyxia can cause you to act irrationally and become a danger to yourself or others. The special safety concerns involved in scuba diving are beyond the scope of this book, but are completely covered in the required coursework for becoming a certified scuba diver. High-altitude mountaineering, skydiving, and other activities whereby you might find yourself at extremely high altitudes, also require coursework and training before you can enter their potentially dangerous domains. There are many specific safety considerations for exercising at extremely high altitude and they, too, are beyond the scope of this book.

But before participating in any potentially dangerous activity, it is advisable that special activity-specific training be taken.

Part 4—What Injuries Teach Us

"How did you become one of the world's most successful people?"
"Good judgment."
"How did you develop such good judgment?"
"Experience."
"How did you gain your wealth of experience?"
"Poor judgment."

Fortunately, even though most of us qualify as "slow learners," we eventually do learn from our mistakes. We learn to recognize potential hazards before crashing into them and develop strategies for avoiding them. We devise methods for coping with our injuries when they do occur in order to minimize them. We learn to pay attention as a means of taking fewer missteps, and we learn to better assess our capabilities so that we put ourselves in jeopardizing situations less frequently.

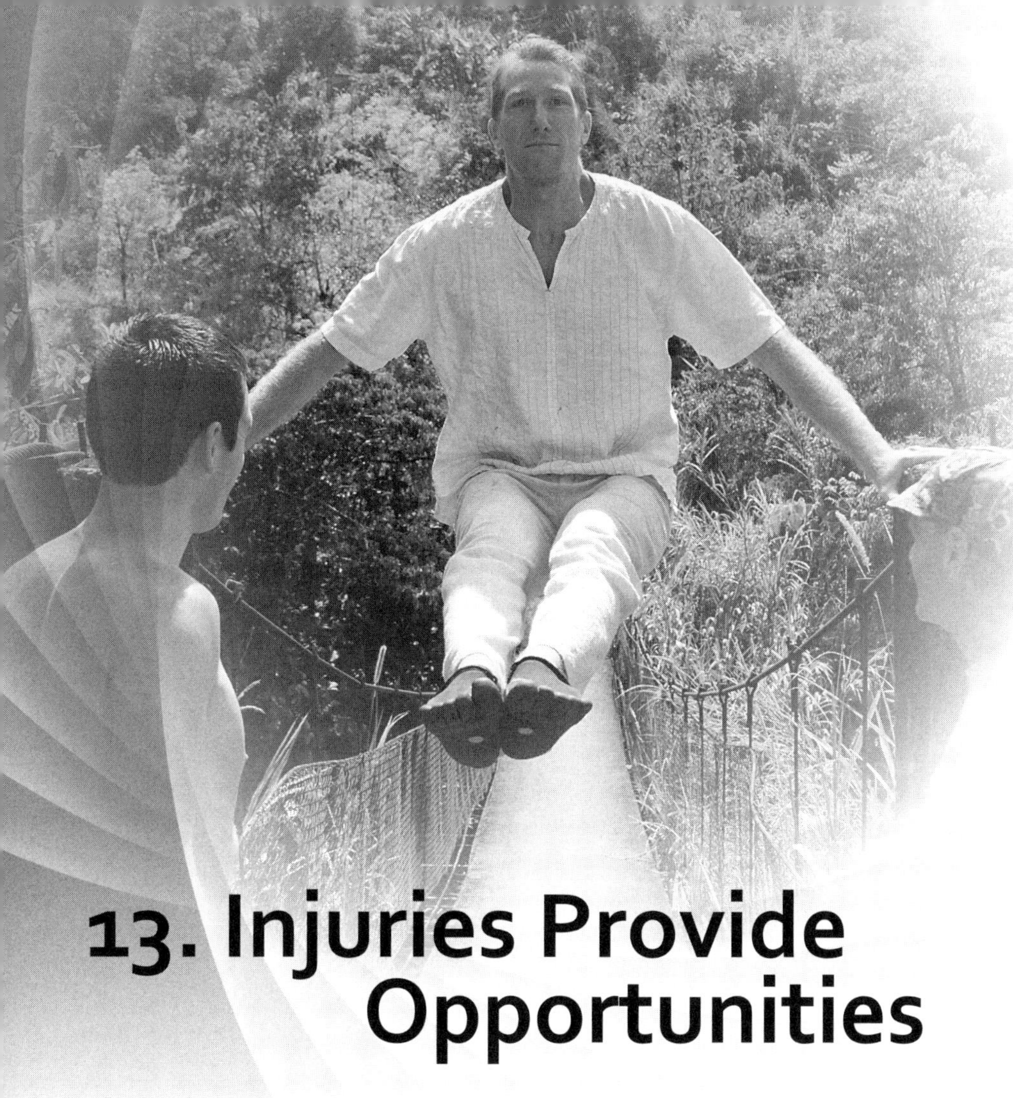

13. Injuries Provide Opportunities

Every event in life can be seen as a blessing, if you choose to see them as such. Even incurring an injury can be seen in a positive light. Likely any injury could have been worse and you now know not to make that same mistake again.

A much-needed update on the value of caution has also been provided. Perhaps most importantly, injuries provide an opportunity to develop aspects of yourself and your fitness performance that have not been given sufficient attention. A broad base of fitness skills is essential if you hope to continually progress in your ability levels. Addressing aspects of training that you usually ignore will help keep you injury-free, while increasing your athletic skills and enjoyment.

A CHANCE TO PRACTICE

With today's improved understanding of well-rounded training principles, interruptions in training are unnecessary if injury does occur. The weight lifter with a bad back, the sprinter with an injured Achilles tendon, the bowler with a vision problem, the dancer with vertigo—all are being held back needlessly.

"Injury provides the opportunity to focus on aspects of training that usually receive insufficient attention."

Injury provides the opportunity to focus on aspects of training that usually receive insufficient attention. There is always *something* athletes can do, regardless of the impediment that seems to be holding them back. Focusing their efforts on undertrained areas in downtime benefits athletes tremendously. A sprained ankle used to mean two weeks or more away from training. Today, an ankle sprain can open the door for flexibility, strength, and neurological training.

Runners are notorious for not doing enough stretching. For the distance runner especially, the excuse is that there simply isn't enough time. When an injury finally occurs, a big gap in the schedule is created, one that used to be filled by running. If inflexibility had anything to do with the injury, the injury provides both the motivation and the time to pay greater attention to flexibility.

There are so many aspects to physical fitness that it is truly difficult to be well-developed in all of them. Usually, we slip into a routine of training, focusing on specific aspects of fitness and forgetting about those that we leave out. Injury often snaps us out of our reveries. If we find that we cannot perform our preferred fitness activities but still want to remain active, there are plenty of alternatives from which to choose.

An injury can give you the time you need to practice aspects of your sport that you could otherwise not find the time for. Many people have developed the desirable quality of being ambidextrous at their sport during a time when their dominant arm was injured. Quite a few gymnasts discovered that they had the potential for extreme flexibility while they were sidelined from other facets of training due to an injury. I personally know of several people who discovered and developed previously unknown talents while pursuing alternate fitness options during their recovery.

DO WHAT YOU LIKE

We are all prone to falling into the following cycles of training: We tend to enjoy doing the things that we are good at. The more we do them, the better we get at them. As we get better, we enjoy them more and subsequently do them more. Those activities that we are not particularly good at often provide us with little more than frustration. We don't enjoy performing them, hence we do not practice them. The less we practice, the worse we become at them. As our specific abilities in weaker areas wane further, we come to like these activities even less, hence we do them still less frequently.

PRACTICE WHAT YOU NEED

The secret to developing well-rounded fitness, or comprehensive abilities in any sport, is to practice those aspects at which you are particularly poor. With more practice, your performance will improve. As your performance level rises, so will your enjoyment. More enjoyment leads to the desire for more practicing. This cycle will repeat itself continually, resulting in an upward spiral of ability and enjoyment. Essentially, if you practice those skills and drills that you like the least, which are also likely the ones you perform poorest, you will get better at them and come to love them. Eventually, you can abolish all weaknesses by turning your weaknesses into strengths.

Getting yourself to practice those skills for which you do not feel you have talent or desire is sometimes a bit of a trick. To do it successfully requires that you focus on bigger goals. Long-term happiness, most people agree, is more important than short-term pleasure. A lifetime of injury-free fitness is more rewarding than a career-ending injury. Fit and healthy for life is more fulfilling than flash-in-the-pan fame.

One of the best feelings in the world is in knowing that *you already did.* Running, cycling, swimming, rowing, and many other activities are fun. People who exercise regularly come to look forward to it, every day. But the best feeling that comes with daily exercise is knowing that you already did yours for the day. Being that satisfied with yourself for a job well-done is an experience that cannot come often enough. Practicing the drills and skills that will serve you throughout your life brings more happiness than wishing you had.

STRENGTHEN YOUR WEAKEST LINK

Stretch a chain until it breaks and you can be pretty darn sure that the link that broke was the weakest one. This same principle holds true for fitness performance and injuries too. If you run faster and faster until you can no longer run, it is likely that either your legs or your lungs will give out. Most people who are not trained runners say that their legs give out first. The runners usually say that it was their lungs—or more specifically, their ability to uptake, transport, and deliver oxygen—and not their legs. Finding someone who says it was a perfect balance of the two is rare. The factor that resulted in the runner having to stop was the weakest link. To achieve better balance and be able to improve performance, emphasis must be placed, at least temporarily, on the weakest aspect of fitness, rather than the strengths. The weak links prevent the strong links from progressing.

If a joint is far more flexible than its surrounding musculature is strong and stabilizing, the cartilage of the joint will be prone to sprain injuries. If the muscles surrounding the joint are exceptionally strong but there is not good flexibility, a muscle or tendon strain will likely be the more common injury incurred. Either way, the imbalance is fostering an increased likelihood for injury.

Most people know their strongest and weakest fitness links. Within any given sport, game, or fitness activity, most people know what they are good and bad at. Making your strengths stronger while ignoring your weak areas does not serve you: this only makes them, and your entire program, weaker. Weak links will hold you back, regardless of your strength. If you have a great tennis serve, it can be a huge asset. But if you cannot hit a backhand well, your serve will not be enough to win matches for you. Once your opponents figure out that you don't have a good backhand, you know they will take advantage of it. It will hold you back incessantly until you improve it.

Why delay putting time into your weakest performance links? They hold you back and increase your risk of injury. They make your overall performance and participation less fun. Putting effort into your weak links will provide you with the opportunity to make the fastest progress with the least amount of exertion.

Let's go back to the "great serve, weak backhand" example. You could practice your great serve for another ten hours and you would not be a much better tennis player, if you improved at all. But put fifteen minutes or half an hour into improving your backhand and you will likely make great strides toward improving it. Remember, your backhand is so bad that it can only get better. To the degree that your backhand improves, so will your overall game. Improve your weakest links: they are the only things holding you back.

How Weak Links Hold You Back

Within your nervous system, you have two types of nerves. One type, sensory nerves, tell you what is going on in the world around you and within you. The other type, motor nerves, send messages to your muscles so that you can respond to your sensory nerve input. Every time you learn a new motor skill, the functioning of all motor pathways improves. Essentially, the motor nerves become increasingly efficient at functioning as you acquire more physical skills. Learning new motor skills is like greasing the skids of motor performance. So if you want to improve your overall physical abilities, learn as many new motor skills as possible; even learning variations of the skills you already know, will help.

The gaps in your physical abilities will show up, and often at the most inopportune times. We already mentioned the tennis player with a poor backhand. Imagine a person that knows how to do a cartwheel but doesn't know how to do a handstand. Now imagine asking that person to perform only the first half of a cartwheel. A cartwheel actually goes through a handstand, and without knowing a handstand, the quality of the cartwheel is diminished. The half-cartwheel will be impossible to perform until a handstand is first learned.

Almost every physical skill can be learned in progressions that are rooted in fundamental movement patterns. These basic movement patterns function as the foundation upon which all the advanced skills are supported. Progressing in any fitness activity is like building a pyramid. The larger the base of support, the higher you can go in learning advanced skills. If any of the basics are missing, it will show up as limitations in overall learning capacity. When people attempt to learn specific advanced skills without taking the time to learn and master all of the basics upon which the advanced skill is rooted, they expose themselves to likely injury. When we watch them in their efforts, the movements do not look smooth, and sometimes, may even look dangerous.

A skier with poor fundamentals may be able to survive while coming down a beginner slope, but there will be extraneous and even wild movements of the arms, legs, and body that indicate lack of control. A skier with good fundamentals should be able to come down the same slope perfectly, with not even one break in form. Put both of those skiers on an intermediate slope, and the skier with poor fundamentals will likely be able to ski down (albeit with a few falls and without control) while the skier with solid fundamentals will sail down the slope without a hitch.

Whereas a good skier can link controlled turns, one after the next, a skier who lacks basics is described as "linking one loss of control with the next." As the mechanical stress imposed by the steepness of the slope increases, the likelihood of falls and injuries rises for the skier with poor or missing basic movement elements. In the high-stress mechanics required for racing through gates or skiing down steep slopes, a lack of basics results in a loss of control every time. The likelihood of injury in every fitness activity increases dramatically if any of the beginner skills are missing from your repertoire. Take the time to learn the basics, however long it requires, for it is well worth your effort.

MAKE FRIENDS WITH THE ENEMY

"Please don't throw me in the briar patch." ~ Br'er Rabbit

Every fitness activity has at least one aspect that you will find more challenging than the others. A decathlete may be able to perform all ten skills required in the decathlon, but will invariably have a favorite and least-favorite one. I worked recently with a professional triathlete, a man who swims, rides his bicycle, and runs for a living. He is an excellent runner, is talented on the bike, but is weak in swimming. Weak, that is, compared to his competition.

I suggested to him that if he wanted to improve his overall times, since total elapsed time is the only one that really matters in a triathlon, he would do best to put more effort into his swimming. He thought otherwise. He said that since he only "loses" about eight minutes on the swim, he would be better off to keep improving his running and swimming in order to "make up" those minutes. He felt that the time spent improving his swimming technique would take too much time and effort away from his running and cycling.

Eight minutes is a lot of time to give up in a race, even in a race that lasts eight hours. The swimming issue had nothing to do with fitness, we both agreed, but had to do solely with technique. Bicycling also requires good technique, but swimming is the most technical of the three activities of the triathlon. By simply taking a few minutes, or even a few hours, to improve technique, I explained, he could speed his swimming for the rest of his career. He saw the logic and agreed.

MAXIMIZED PROGRESS

If you were going to live forever, there would be no urgency in any of your self-improvement goals. You could take your time when learning new skills, converting weaknesses to strengths, and developing healthier habits. But then, of course, if you were going to live forever, healthy habits might not interest you. Though the likelihood of living forever is slim, knowing this gives a certain sweet urgency to all that we do. Time races on, and as we grow in age, so often do we also grow in our desire to take better care of ourselves. Efficient and effective progress in all aspects of life, especially our health and fitness care, becomes increasingly essential.

Streamlining the day's activities to eliminate extraneous and wasted effort becomes ever more important. While smelling the roses along the way is also an integral part of healthful living, the bottom line, or return on investment, also is a primary consideration. In any field of endeavor, and certainly in exercise and sports performance, we all want to learn how to make the most progress with the least amount of effort.

The downtime that accompanies an injury can be the most severe interruption of training that we ever incur. When we aren't practicing those skills that we love on a regular basis, we are losing them. Though injuries provide us with opportunity to practice skills that we might otherwise ignore, and though they sometimes open doors for us that result in an overall improvement in performance, they definitely result in certain types of setbacks as well.

Any time that an injury can be avoided, it should be. Still, it is likely that an active person will now and then experience some sort of injury, no matter how minor. The following are ideas for training that will reduce the downtime incurred by injury to the absolute minimum.

PREHABILITATION

Every physical pursuit has its own specific injury propensities. If you are a hiker, for instance, you are more likely to injure your foot, ankle, knee, or leg, than your arm. Some sports even have commonly incurred injuries or conditions named after them: tennis elbow, surfer's knee, golfer's elbow, and swimmer's ear, to name just a few. In every field of physical endeavor, certain types of injuries can almost be predicted.

Basketball players twist their ankles, gymnasts get blisters on their hands, football players injure their knees, dancers develop sore feet, sprinters tear their hamstrings, baseball pitchers damage their shoulders, and low-back injuries plague almost everyone. Knowing the type of injury to which your chosen activity predisposes you can help you to prevent it from occurring. Knowing this can also encourage you to prepare for the injury's eventuality by doing the appropriate exercises that will make rehabilitation easier and faster.

"Whatever the activity or the injury likely to accompany it, it is possible to prehabilitate yourself."

Rehabilitation is the term used to describe the activities, exercises, and education that is used in recovering from an injury or surgery. The word "prehabilitation" refers to the activities, exercises, and education that one undergoes *before* incurring an injury or surgery. My niece, a world-class softball pitcher, injured her shoulder and required corrective surgery.

The doctors explained that she would require three months of specific exercises for her rehabilitation before she could resume normal activities. As the surgery was scheduled three months in advance, I encouraged her to begin her exercise program for the shoulder immediately. She did prehabilitation exercises for three months. After the surgery, her rehabilitation exercises went extremely well. They were almost easy for her, as she had done so much in preparation for them, and she recovered much more rapidly than predicted.

If your chosen activity is one that often results in ankle sprains, it is a good idea to do prehabilitation on your ankles before ever having a problem. Whatever the activity or the injury likely to accompany it, it is possible to prehabilitate yourself.

What is not possible, however, is to be prepared for every possible injury in any given physical pursuit. Accidents happen, and they cannot always be predicted. Prehabilitation is an excellent way of diminishing the likelihood of the occurrence of those injuries that can be predicted, and of reducing the downtime from them should they actually happen anyway.

Time Best Spent

I had a client who repeatedly suffered from ankle sprains, three to four times per year, minimum. He would wear ankle braces if he suspected that he was about to participate in an "ankle unfriendly" activity, but found that he often would sprain an ankle even at other times. He realized that he was spending weeks, and sometimes months, out of every year, recovering from ankle sprains. He noticed that he was also becoming less willing to participate in activities that challenged his ankles, even though he loved sports such as tennis, basketball, and squash.

I suggested to him that his time would be best spent doing prehabilitation for his ankles. I showed him the proper exercises for strengthening all of the musculature that supported his ankles. I taught him the drills that would improve his reflexes and give him the proper responses to any situation where his ankle would begin to twist. In a few sessions with me, he learned the related postural skills, so that he would no longer be as likely to put his ankles into vulnerable positions when standing, walking, running, jumping, or changing direction.

We worked on his balance, and corrected imbalances, so that his ankles would be subjected to less mechanical stress when he played sports. After just a few weeks of working together, he felt far more confident. Over the next ten years, instead of twisting his ankle thirty or forty more times, as he would have expected, he only experienced a total of three ankle sprains, and none had been in the last five years.

There is an old saying, whose author is unknown: "You've got to do what you've got to do in order to get what you want to get." If you keep finding that certain injuries are holding you back, it is time well spent to learn and practice the preventive measures.

Rarely does anyone find prehabilitation or rehabilitation to be fun, but they beat getting injured. Although prehabilitation exercises can be a bit repetitious and tedious, they can be structured to be fun, too. Your attitude makes the biggest difference in that regard. You'll make far better use of your time by spending an hour or two in specific prehabilitative exercises to avoid an injury than you would by spending weeks or months in rehabilitation for that same injury.

EFFICIENT AND EFFECTIVE COMPREHENSIVE REHABILITATION

Efficient rehabilitative procedures bring about the desired results in the shortest amount of time with the least amount of effort. Effective ones do exactly the job that needed doing, and well enough so that it does not have to be done again. When rehabilitating any part of the body after an injury or surgery, all five aspects of fitness performance need to be considered. The injured part should be able to withstand the stresses of training for cardiopulmonary, muscular strength, muscular endurance, flexibility, and neurological abilities by the time that rehabilitation is completed. If the rehabilitation is not comprehensive, it leaves the door wide open for reinjury.

The efficient rehabilitation program is extremely focused. While each case must be considered on an individual basis, the same rules of training apply to rehabilitation as they do for regular fitness sessions. Warm-up, train, and cool-down as always. Apply a reasonable degree of overload, using frequency, intensity, and duration as variables to stimulate the training effect.

Allow plenty of time for all of the lifestyle necessities that encourage optimum recovery. Vary your training sufficiently to keep it fresh, fun, and interesting. Use prehabilitation procedures to prevent the onset of another injury.

Effective rehabilitation is always focused on the goal of eliminating the need for further rehabilitation. All drills, skills, and training during rehabilitation must relate in some way to the repair and maintenance of the injured part. There is pressure on many physical therapists to perform their training as rapidly as possible.

Cutting corners can allow someone to finish their rehabilitation more rapidly, but cutting corners invariably leads to a subsequent injury that is often more severe than the original. Ask your therapists about every exercise, and how it relates to your rehabilitation. The more focused you both stay in your sessions, the faster you can be done with your rehabilitation.

REHABILITATION FOR SPRAINS AND DISLOCATIONS

Fortunately, there are several effective methods for rehabilitating the ankles and avoiding ankle injuries. Strength is part of the picture, as is correcting the body mechanics that may lead to subsequent sprains. But top on the list is the "proprioception board," or balance board, as they are commonly known.

This board is designed to provide an unstable platform, but with adjustable limits to the board's range of motion so that the amount of instability can be controlled. With practice, one can learn to react more rapidly, and correctly, to a situation that is potentially dangerous to the ankle. Eventually, ankle sprains can become a thing of the past, even for people with "weak" ankles.

FOOL ME ONCE...

Injuries happen, usually unexpectedly, and that is the danger of getting out of bed. Nonetheless, we all do it if we can. From the most methodical safety enthusiasts to the wildest of the thrill seekers, we all want to experience physical activity. Most thrill seekers, in fact, will tell you that they are taking well-calculated risks, and that they in no way expect or intend to get hurt, even during their most daring stunts. They simply find that pushing their physical and mental limits to the maximum is interesting—like nothing else they can do. They really like paying attention.

Many other people actually choose their fitness activity because they don't have to pay attention while performing it. Their high-stress job demands all the attention they care to give for the day. Riding an exercise bike, running on a treadmill, or rowing a machine gives them a physical outlet while mentally they can simply "space out" for a while. Either way, or anywhere in between, accidents still happen. The trick is not to let the same accident happen more than once. There is no end of accidents just waiting to happen.

Life has a way of teaching us lessons. When we learn a lesson, it is replaced by another. There will always be another lesson. As of yet, no one has learned them all, at least to my knowledge. If you do not learn your lesson the first time it is brought to you, it will be brought to you again and again, in an ever more powerful form. Eventually, we either learn the lesson or we get crushed by it.

"Most thrill seekers find that pushing their physical and mental limits to the maximum is interesting like nothing else they can do."

Nature's lessons are quite straightforward. The laws of nature are immutable; they cannot be broken. You can prove them, but you cannot break them. These laws, such as the law of gravity, are always in effect. There is no "time-out." If you try to break a law of nature, Nature will break you. We typically learn to respect the laws of nature rather early in life, though often as teenagers we forget, and we have to learn that respect again. There is no dishonor in making mistakes. There is great honor in learning from them.

REPEAT INJURIES

As a kid, I hit my thumb with a hammer a couple of times. I try not to do that anymore. I am more cautious about how I hold the nail, and how I swing the hammer. I might be a bit more meticulous these days, but I get hurt a lot less often. I spend less time laid up with injuries and because of it I get a lot more done overall, meticulous as I may be. Repeating the same old injury is never a point of pride.

"Repeat injuries simply need not happen. If they do, learn the lesson and change something in your approach to that activity."

More often than not, repeat injuries happen because people do bad or harmful things to themselves. If you hit your thumb with a hammer a few times while building several houses, you would never point to your thumb and say, "I have a bad thumb that's been giving me a lot of trouble lately. It acts up with no provocation." The reality is that the thumb was fine until it was abused.

The thumb is a good thumb. If it didn't hurt when it was hit with a hammer, there would be something wrong with it indeed. Yet people will quickly say, "I have a bad back," or, "I have a bad stomach," when in actuality they had to treat those parts rather harshly in order for them to complain. Repeat injuries are essentially a sign of body abuse. Develop a loving relationship with your body.

Give it the rehabilitation it needs in order to thrive. Once thriving, give it the prehabilitation it deserves, and all of the healthful conditions it requires. Repeat injuries simply need not happen. If they do, learn the lesson and change something in your approach to that activity.

FINISHING THE JOB

When I was a teenager, a friend's father hurt his back. I saw him one day, diligently doing exercises in his bedroom. "It was terrible," he said. "The pain was so severe that I was totally bedridden. I never intend to hurt my back again. I will do these exercises every day, for the rest of my life." When I was in my mid-twenties, I too hurt my back, and it was humbling. I did the requisite exercises, but only for a short while. A pattern developed where I would injure myself, feel terrible, do the exercises, feel better, stop doing the exercises, and eventually reinjure myself. Ten years passed before I committed to doing the exercises every day for the rest of my life. They only take about two minutes per day.

The temptation to get back into your chosen physical activity after an injury can be very strong, but this must be tempered by the reality of not wanting to reinjure yourself. Going back to running, tennis, or whatever activity you injured yourself playing too soon, will usually have disastrous results. Incurring the same injury, or even a different one, is simply not worth the time it takes in recovery, especially if waiting just a few more days would have made all the difference in the world. Pay attention to the finishing details of recovery. Make sure that you are 100 percent ready to go before you go 100 percent all-out.

"Incurring the same injury, or even a different one, is simply not worth the time it takes in recovery, especially if waiting just a few more days would have made all the difference in the world."

NEW EYES

You may think that you are recovering well from a certain injury. Perhaps you hurt your knee, and had to limp for a while. Eventually, you can walk normally, and even carefully go up and down stairs. As you progress, your knee gains the ability to bear weight and the spring in your step returns. Soon enough, you feel completely healed, and you go out to play with people who have maintained their ability level (your previous one), while yours declined. When you see how easily they move, you realize that you still have a while to go till you are fully recovered. It's like seeing yourself through new eyes.

Get an outside opinion on your recovery progress after an injury. There is no advantage in trying to do it all yourself. Second and third opinions can prove extremely valuable. Often, other people can add their experience to yours, broadening your scope of understanding about what happened to you and what you can do about it. A team of supporters can give you perspective and insight that you might never have been able to have achieved on your own. Utilize the services of new eyes whenever you can. The input of professionals, as well as that of amateurs, may make all the difference between a successfully finished rehabilitation and an incomplete one.

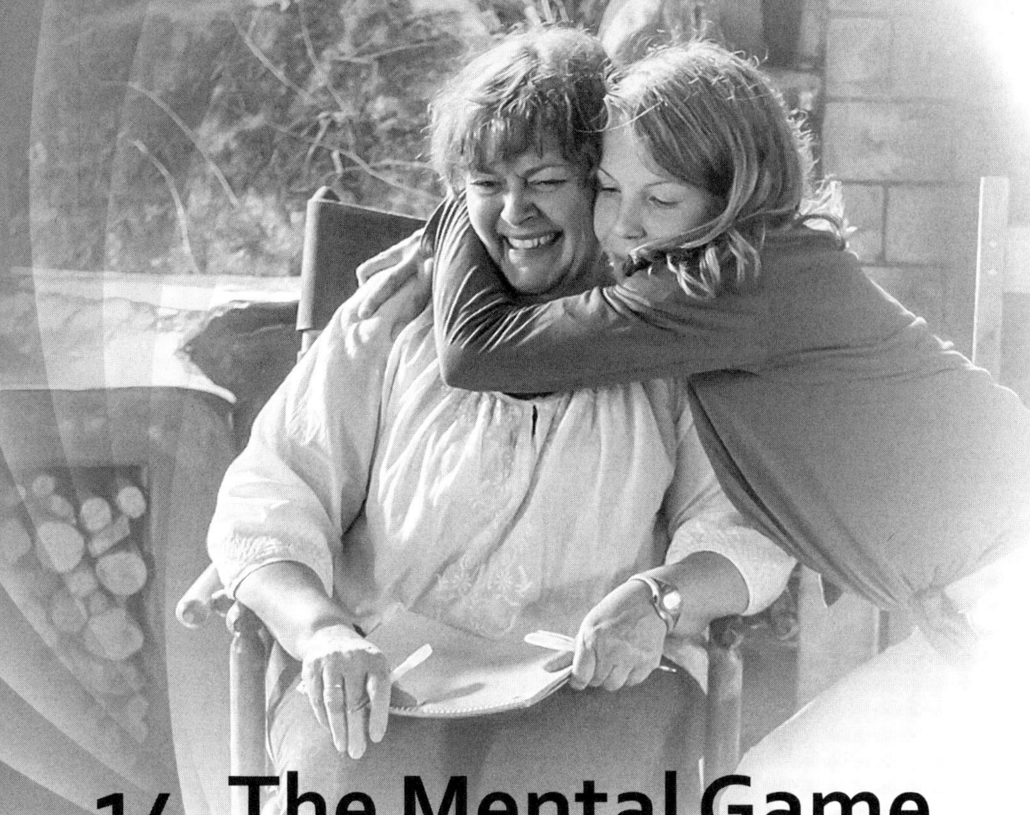

14. The Mental Game

"Winners never quit and quitters never win." ~Anonymous

Little injuries are usually insignificant. They represent minor inconveniences, small setbacks, and nothing more. Often enough, you will consider these injuries as unimportant, or not even consider them at all. The modest impact of such accidents can realistically be ranked as inconsequential in the bigger scheme of things. Rarely does such physical damage warrant a second thought, as the impairment, if any, is very short-lived and recovery is taken for granted.

With a small cut, bruise, scrape, or tear, or even with a broken bone, the healing experience is relatively commonplace. We know the healing time involved and we know we are going to get completely well. When looking into the future, it is easy to see beyond the injury to a time when we will be whole again. We hold this vision that in our mind as we go through the process of healing.

We can't always see the end of an injury, however. It can be extremely challenging, mentally, to feel that we are in the midst of something that

"We can't always see the end of an injury, however. It can be extremely challenging, mentally, to feel that we are in the midst of something that might never end."

might never end. The function of every cell of our body is affected by what we think. Accepting permanent impairment, even as a possibility, is completely different physiologically than expecting complete recovery. Coming up with a healthy way of dealing with the idealism of hope, the realism of honesty, and the bleakness of depression that can accompany a serious injury is a serious juggling act.

INJURIES CAN BE DEVASTATING

The physical pain associated with most sports and exercise injuries, even the more severe ones, is relatively short in duration. It is the mental anguish we experience that can really last. The degree of emotional discomfort can become overwhelming and cause some people to give up hope for recovery. The impact of injury on the psyche can be huge. Our will to persist in developing our physical abilities is a mental decision.

We all experience setbacks now and then. Usually we overcome them, or find a way around them. "Every man has his breaking point," or so it is said. Far too many people have given up their childhood dreams of being fit and healthy throughout their lives. Many of those people gave up after incurring a serious injury they couldn't imagine themselves ever fully recovering from.

We must keep looking forward, focus on solutions instead of problems, and to envision ourselves as whole, healthy, and useful individuals. I am not suggesting that we ignore reality, but that we insist on always putting our best foot forward.

There is an old saying, "When I see it, I will believe it," meaning that we must be shown before we can believe. I think that the opposite is true; that by believing something you can help to make it become a reality. The human will can be the most powerful force on earth. Keep your will focused on recovery and it cannot be distracted by any obstacle.

NEVER AGAIN?

If you fall off your horse, bicycle, or skis, conventional wisdom says that it is important that you get right back "in the saddle" and prove to yourself that you still can do it. If not, it is said that your mental image of the fall will likely grow in size, disproportionate to the actual event, and you may become afraid to ever try your hand at that activity again.

Your fears may even grow to where you won't try other activities that you see as related to or associated with the initial one. There is a great deal of truth in this age-old advice. We will discuss fear in more depth later in this chapter.

DEALING WITH LETDOWNS...NEXT

There are many times during the course of each day that we must deal with letdowns. They are a fact of life. Most of the little disappointments go by without notice, but in fact we deal with them in exactly the same way that we can successfully deal with the big ones. We cope with the small frustrations so efficiently that we often don't even really know how we did it.

If someone were to ask, "What was your strategy for handling that problem?" in reference to a really small issue, your likely first answer would be, "I don't know," because you did it automatically, without thinking. We simply pay more attention to the big issues. We consider them, put a lot of thought into them, and often make them more difficult to deal with than they truly are.

What is this automatic success strategy that we use intuitively with the little issues of life? With the little things, we simply say, "next." Then we move on, and do whatever it is that truly is next. With bigger issues such as a serious injury, the solution is just as simple. Since there is no going back in time, the only realistic solution is to say, "NEXT." (Since this is a bigger issue, it rightfully deserves a bigger "next.")

Accepting that the injury happened is not the same thing as accepting that the disability it incurs is permanent. Acceptance is simply a step toward assessing the damage and implementing the correction. Until you say, "NEXT" and really mean it, however, you will be stuck: powerless in the past.

CREATING THE NEWEST SCHEDULE

"Congratulate yourself as you go, realizing that every step is a step closer to your destination."

With a realistic assessment of your current status and your willingness to move forward from your injury confirmed by your sincere decree of "NEXT," it is time to create a new training schedule. One of the most uplifting experiences any human can have is to overcome an obstacle. The creation of a new training schedule, therefore, should be a celebratory event. Exciting times are ahead and there is much progress to be made.

Unfulfilled expectations can be quite a letdown. Still, goals need a time limit. In order to avoid the frustration of falling short on a goal, make your goals realistic and resettable. Make the goal realistic, and you will likely achieve it in the time frame you have set for yourself. If you do not reach your goal in the predetermined time frame, reassess the situation and reset the goal, giving it a future date of completion.

Achieving a goal can be incredibly rewarding, and failing to attain them can be equally frustrating. Coming back from an injury is challenging enough without having to deal with the frustration of falling short of your goals. In order to diminish the likelihood of not meeting your goals, break them down into the smallest component parts that you can. Let the goals build, one on top of another, rather than simply reaching for the endpoint. Congratulate yourself as you go, realizing that every step is a step closer to your destination.

HE SAYS... SHE SAYS...

I was friends and business partners with a married couple named Ron and Babs Camp in the early eighties. They were wonderful people who taught me a lot. Ron was famous for his sayings, most notably, "Plan your work and work your plan." He never quit, and never admitted to losing. He coached a football team for 15 years and of that time he said, "We never lost a game. We ran out of time now and again, but we never lost."

Babs supplied Ron's balance in life. She worked with him, and as hard as he did too. She was amazingly good with people, somehow always making everyone feel at ease. Her motto was, "Make plans, be flexible." The reality of life is that both mottoes are necessary, each in their own time.

RISE UP WITH ROLE MODELS

Many people are self-motivated, but all of us respond well to the people we look up to. We will often do more for someone else than we will do for ourselves. Whether we want to impress them, imitate them, or simply to learn from them, role models have what we need. No one person can have or be everything for you. You may aspire to have the business acumen of one person, the athleticism of another, and the people skills of yet another.

In sports, you might want to be able to duplicate one person's powerful start, someone else's consistency, and a third person's kick at the finish. These people might even come from different sports. Whatever the skills you are hoping to learn, you can learn them the fastest from someone who already has them. You can get what you want from the people who have it and those people should become your role models.

AIN'T SO BAD

One of the most inspirational sports stories of all time is exemplified in the *Rocky* movie series. Rocky overcame one obstacle after another, winning against what seemed like impossible odds. When things got tough and Rocky started to really feel the pressure of impending defeat, his famous line was, "You ain't so bad." Once he had convinced himself that the current challenge he was facing wasn't so bad, he knew that he could overcome it. By telling his opponents "You ain't so bad," he got them to believe it too.

If you tell yourself that something is impossible, it probably is. If you convince yourself that something is achievable, it probably is too. When we look at what others have achieved, and see how they have risen to the top of their chosen field, it makes it that much easier for us to rise with them.

Use role models for your motivation. Read the stories of the underdogs who have gone on to make it big. Almost any mountain would seem hard to climb if you were the first one to climb it. But if you know that hundreds of others have already gone there before you, there is no reason why you cannot reach the peak as well. Let your role models serve to give you a hand up.

YOU'VE GOT TO HAVE HEROES

In the world of sports there have been some amazing people. There are more brilliant sports stories, true stories, than you could ever read in a lifetime. Glenn Cunningham was severely burned in a fire as a child. He was expected to die and was told that if he lived he would never walk. He went on to hold the world record in the mile run.

Although now tainted by scandal, O. J. Simpson overcame huge obstacles to become a star football player. He was born deformed, and his parents were told he would never walk. Through perseverance, he transformed himself into one of the greatest running backs in American football history. Such stories of overcoming obstacles could fill a book. Learn about these people and let them motivate you to strive for and achieve great things.

Sports heroes come in many types. Some are considered great for their physical accomplishments. Others rise to greatness because besides being super athletes, they are wonderful people. Some make a habit of regularly visiting children in hospitals. Some quit their sports at the height of their careers to follow a higher calling. Some perform their best when the odds are most against them, or they always seem to come through with clutch and last-minute performances. Whoever your heroes are, and for whatever reason you hold them in high regard, know that when you are looking up you have the greatest chance of rising up. People who have trained against their heroes, even if only mentally, have registered some of the best performances ever

"If you tell yourself that something is impossible, it probably is. If you convince yourself that something is achievable, it probably is too."

achieved. These heroes made them continually raise the bar toward and beyond the known limits.

STRIVE TO MAKE SOMEONE PROUD

Children love to be watched. Often a child who seems totally engrossed in play will stop and look up, just to see if mom or dad is watching. If you need more motivation to stay with your rehabilitation program, make use of the people who care the most about you. They want to see you happy, to see you succeed. Do it for them. Each day, as you decide whether to go through with another day of training, think about the people who would be proud of you for doing it. When you are wondering if training is worth the effort, imagine yourself accepting the praise of someone you really care about. Even if it all happens just inside your own head, you will find that striving to imbue someone with a good opinion of you will prove supremely motivational.

EMOTIONALLY READY FOR INJURY?

There is only so much that you can do to prepare yourself for having an injury. The prehabilitation concept helps you physically, both to prevent injury and in the case that one does still happen. But being emotionally prepared is another story altogether. Accidents are unexpected, that is part of their nature. How can you prepare for the unexpected? About the only thing that you can count on is that if an accident is going to happen, it will likely happen at such a time and in such a fashion as to cause you the most possible inconvenience.

INJURY IS A REAL RISK

Physical activities of all types include risk as part and parcel of participation. Sometimes it is even dangerous to be a spectator. Although no one starts a fitness program expecting to get hurt, it would be unwise to pretend that injury is simply not a possibility. By taking proper precautions such as wearing protective gear, performing appropriate warm-up and cool-down skills, taking classes where indicated, and participating at a difficulty level that matches your abilities, you can at least minimize your risks. Since the overall health risks of the sedentary life are greater than those of being fit, safely participating in exercise is actually the safest move you can make.

TAKING GREAT CARE OF YOURSELF IS EASY WHEN ALL IS GOING WELL

> **"One of the challenges to staying healthy and fit for a lifetime is that life intervenes in unexpected ways."**

One of the challenges to staying healthy and fit for a lifetime is that life intervenes in unexpected ways. When you are living according to your schedule and everything is going according to plan, it is relatively easy to take great care of yourself. But when unexpected events happen and you become stressed, they sometimes seem to almost force you to break your schedule. If fitness is viewed as a chore to perform and you are running late due to an unexpected traffic jam, your fitness program might be squeezed out of the schedule. If fitness is viewed as a treat, then you will find time for it even if it means that dinner will be a little later than usual.

Normally you may follow your diet plan perfectly. But on a high-stress day you may feel the temptation to eat or drink "comfort foods" that are not usually on your menu. However, the time to take the best care of yourself is when you are stressed. In the same way that you would nurture a child having a hard time, nurture yourself when things get rough.

Be extra kind to yourself when you feel life's stress. Eat extra well. Give yourself more time to train than usual. Go to bed an hour early. Knowing that you are most vulnerable to falling off your fitness plan when times are stressful, and that keeping up your exercise program will help with stress reduction, will give you that much more incentive to stay regular with your training.

HAVE YOUR "B PLAN" READY

If you normally work out every morning but lately just haven't had the time, have you been getting in your training at midday instead?

Do you keep an extra pair of sneakers and some workout gear in your car or at work, just in case a fitness opportunity arises? If you can't get to the gym to do your normal strength-training routine because it's closed for repairs for eight weeks, do you know how to strength train at home? Do you have the necessary equipment, or know how to do it without equipment? If your squash or tennis partner simply fails to show up, do you go home or do you have a "B plan"? Always have an alternate option for fitness activities. If you are so attached to one specific workout that you cannot enjoy yourself doing anything else, you may have a problem, and need to look at that issue more closely. If you are truly motivated to stay fit, you should always keep your exercise options open.

FEAR, REAL AND IMAGINED

Fear can do funny things to a person. You are more likely to get hurt from acting out of fear and trying to avoid getting hurt than if you just acted naturally. Once you start thinking about what you are doing instead of just doing it, the movements become awkward. Fear is fear, and the person experiencing it doesn't care if it's based on sound logic or imagination.

Fear Can Make You Dangerous to Yourself (and Others)

Once fear comes into play, you start to think too much and perform less efficiently. Let's say you are trying to learn a backward somersault on a trampoline, but are fearful that you are going to land on your head. You have mastered all of the lead-up skills, having done all of them hundreds of times.

The big day arrives, and you have been playing it up, all out of proportion. Your instructor assures you that you are ready, and that he will spot you flawlessly. He says that he will practically be doing the darn thing for you. Yet something inside of you gets dizzy, and you lose almost all sense of perception when you even start thinking about that first backward somersault. Epinephrine is released from the adrenal glands, stimulating the pancreas to send insulin to the bloodstream. The muscles become hyperresponsive as the "flight or fight" response kicks in, raising sensory nerve function to the maximum.

Somehow, you manage to complete the somersault, but are so excited afterward that you totally forget what you are doing. The instructor helps you land on your feet and then lets go of you to congratulate you. Your momentum, which normally you would have the presence of mind to have stopped, carries you backward. You fall down and come very close to getting injured.

An alternative to the above situation might have gone like this: As you prepare to backward somersault, fear so overwhelms you that you come out of your tuck position, spreading your arms and legs wide apart. This not only kills your momentum, but you poke your instructor in the eye with your thumb. He manages to turn you over enough so that you land safely on your hands and knees, but goes home with a black eye nonetheless.

How Fear Delays Recovery from Injury

The major issue regarding fear and recovery is that many people become afraid to test the injured part, for fear that they are going to injure it again. Many people will baby their injury during rehabilitation for this reason. While this makes sense to a degree, it can easily be taken too far. Once fear becomes the major deciding factor in exercise decisions rather than feedback from your body, you have lost control of the situation.

In order to maximize your recovery rate, the training effect must be induced. Fear of injury from exertion can hold you back so far that the training effect is inhibited, slowing recovery radically. At this point, the fear becomes a self-fulfilling prophecy. Not only is rehabilitation slowed, but body mechanics must be compromised to compensate for the injured part. Poor mechanics increase the possibility of future injury, while decreased intensity of training results in an overall decay

"Fear of injury from exertion can hold you back so far that the training effect is inhibited, slowing recovery radically."

in all five aspects of training, increasing the chance of injury yet again. Recovery must be undertaken in a safe and systematic manner. This was discussed in depth in Chapter 6.

WHAT ARE YOU TELLING YOURSELF?

When your mind talks, every cell of your body listens. It's possible to intentionally think thoughts that affect your physiology. Yogis have been known to slow their heart rate dramatically, to raise their body temperature, and to lower their blood pressure, simply through mind control. We all have an impact on our physiological functions through our thoughts, whether intentional or not. There are many books that explain the relationship of our thoughts to our health. Authors such as Louise Hay have explained that it is not only disease, but injuries that are often created through our thoughts. The specific body part affected by the injury can apparently be related to the type of thoughts, as well.

POSTURAL BIOFEEDBACK

The basketball players were running up and down the court, playing a practice game that I was coaching. One player was trying to prove himself, but he was struggling. Almost every time he touched the ball, he would make an error. A missed shot, an errant pass, a loss of ball control; he just couldn't seem to get it right. After every error his head would drop forward, his shoulders would sag, and he would give every appearance of having given up. I called for a break in the action in order to talk things over.

I asked the players to walk the length of the court with their eyes closed, while I talked to them. All I asked them to do was to feel what I was describing. I described them missing a critical shot, losing the game, throwing an embarrassingly bad pass, and in other ways letting down their fans, teammates, coaches, and themselves. As they walked, their posture made it clear that they were listening and feeling. They hung, slumped, drooped, and dragged like defeated men.

On the walk back, I described the opposite scenario, again simply asking them to feel my words. I told them that they had made a crucial play, sunk a difficult shot, and shown court awareness that had saved the day and won the game. As the men walked, they became noticeably taller. They held their heads high, chests out, shoulders broadened. A spring came into their steps. They even smiled. It was truly amazing.

After the drill was completed, I asked the players to simply hold those positive thoughts and that winning posture throughout the rest of the practice. The level of play soared dramatically. The player that was struggling was suddenly on fire; he could do no wrong. When he made an error, it didn't show at all. He remained in the moment, obviously expecting that the very next time he touched the ball was going to be "his" moment.

In order to perform your best you have to think, move, carry yourself, and take care of yourself as if you expect to do your best.

NEURO-LINGUISTIC PROGRAMMING

Neuro-linguistic programming is a version of self-talk. Not only does your posture affect how your body performs, so do your words. Apparently your brain really believes you when you talk, and creates the appropriate reality. If you say, "I am always getting hurt," you are likely going to continue that behavior pattern. If instead you say, "I used to always get hurt but I have put that into my past," there is a good chance that you will reduce your frequency of getting injured. If you tell yourself you are going to fail, you have increased your chances of doing so.

Many Olympic champions mention that they practiced "seeing" themselves having already won the medal, standing on the podium, giving the interviews, and going home and receiving accolades of their friends, family, and nation. They literally talked themselves into winning.

The mind also pays no attention to negative phrasing. If you say to yourself, for instance, "I am not going to miss this shot," the mind omits the word, "not." The same thing will happen if you are trying to learn to ice skate and say, "I will not fall down." Your brain envisions positive action, and creates its constructs accordingly. Use the power of positive action when talking to yourself and others. Phrases such as, "I will make this shot" and "I will stay up," will take you towards your goal. They will make recovery from injury far more efficient and much more effective.

"Use the power of positive action when talking to yourself and others."

OTHER SELF-CONSTRUCTIVE SAFETY METHODS

The same lifestyle factors that make for optimum training conditions make for optimum recovery. Sufficient rest and sleep, fresh air, daylight and sunlight, emotional poise, pure water, fruits and vegetables, positive mental attitude, and regular exercise, all play a role in making recovery speedy and safe.

Extending your warm-up and cool-down is a great idea for making recovery from injury safer. If there is even a chance of reinjury, wearing extra protective gear is also recommended. Choose activities wisely when going through rehabilitation, opting for the ones that offer the least chance for damaging your recovering part(s). If your injury is not visible and obvious, and you are playing with other people, be sure to tell them about it so that they do not bump or hit it inadvertently.

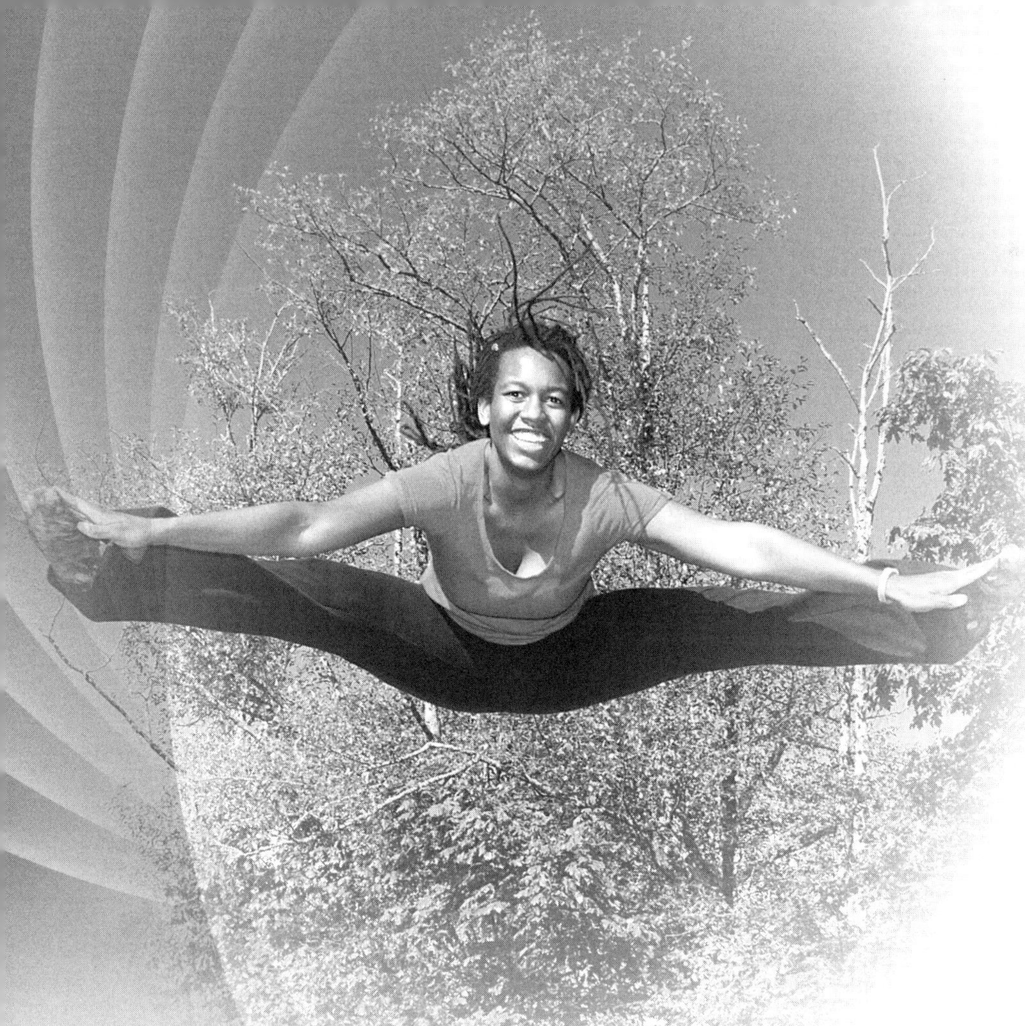

15. Rebirth: Coming Back from Injury

An injury is not a death sentence, and even a relatively serious injury usually does not mean there will be a permanent disability. Most people recover from most injuries as if nothing had ever happened. The following guidelines describe the tactics and techniques used by professional trainers and top athletes when planning their comeback from injury.

BASIC GUIDELINES

Every situation is unique, both in terms of the strengths and weaknesses of the individual and the exact nature of the injury. There are certain guides that will work for everyone, as they use concepts that are universally applicable. Be sure to follow these general guidelines as you design your specific training and rehabilitation program.

SIMULATION

Simulation is the single most powerful training tool available to you. We will mention just a few of the ways it can be used here. Feel free to be creative and invent other methods of putting this tool to use.

Any aspect of training or competition can be simulated in order to gain familiarity with it or to see how you will respond to it. Modifications and adjustments can be made as needed when simulating, something we cannot do in real-life competitions. For purposes of recovery from injury, we primarily want to use simulation to create situations that might stress the injured part, or result in more damage to the injury. We can alter the simulation so that we experience it smaller, slower, in a more focused way, or in some way less stressfully than it would be in reality. This gives us the chance to test the injured part to be sure it is functional and that it won't break down under pressure.

Competition situations can be simulated without introducing the stress of all-out performance or the nervous jitters that often accompany meets or game day. You may be able to travel to the venue ahead of time and run through your events at 70 percent of normal, then 80 percent, and then 90 percent without losing face or disappointing teammates, testing to make sure that your injury will hold up. Repeated simulations allow the athlete to become familiar with the competition routine.

Stress can be further reduced when you know where and when to eat, what the event location will look like, and so on. The more details that can be simulated, the easier the actual event will become for the athlete. If athletes become comfortable with the entire situation and also know that their injuries can handle the stress of competitive exertions, they are essentially ready to go.

PAIN IS A WARNING

Should you feel pain at any point during a simulation or in a training program, stop exercising. Pain is usually a very good indicator that something is about to go wrong, or has already gone wrong, and that exercising will make it worse. You may find that by stopping, stretching, walking, or just lowering the intensity of your exertions, that the pain quickly goes away. If so, it is likely that you can safely resume exercising. If the pain continues, you have a decision to make. Depending on how far you have progressed in your day's training, you are smart to either choose a different activity; one that doesn't hurt at all, or decide that your workout is over for the day. A substantial percentage of all injuries and reinjuries could have been prevented if people would simply stop attempting to train while they are experiencing workout-related pain.

"Pain is usually a very good indicator that something is about to go wrong, or has already gone wrong, and that exercising will make it worse."

RESPECT YOUR PRE- AND POST-WORKOUT SYMPTOMS

Before your workout begins for the day, it is a good idea to notice how you are feeling. If you are tired, achy, or truly not motivated, it is worth taking these symptoms into account when planning your session. You may decide that you need a nap more than you need to keep pushing yourself. During your warm-up, if a specific part of you is sore or you have an injury that just doesn't feel ready for more stress, adjust the nature of your workout accordingly. You prove nothing by being so hard on yourself that you have a relapse or cause a reinjury. There are times when training harder is not training smarter.

Usually during the cool-down everything feels good, and it's difficult to accurately assess how your weakest links are doing at that time. An hour after the workout, or even two hours later however, your body will talk to you, loudly and clearly. Pay attention at these times. If you are more stiff, sore, tired, achy, or feel an overt pain that you don't usually have, be certain to allow for extra rest in your program. Perhaps even plan for a light day the next day, creating space for optimum recovery.

SPECIFIC CONSIDERATIONS

The specific manner in which a given injury is handled by each physical therapist or other health professional is unique. The nature of the injury as well as the health, fitness, genetic makeup, and expectations of the individual, along many other factors, determine proper handling of each client. Yet within that unique framework are certain basic guidelines that hold true for everyone. Once you learn the basics, you can take a great deal of the guesswork out of rebuilding your fitness after almost any injury. If you understand the principles that the rehabilitative therapist is using on your injury, you can then safely do much of the work on your own to assist the rehabilitation process. The following considerations should not be thought of as a substitute for professional care. They should be used in addition to the professional rehabilitative care that is likely necessary if you have experienced a serious injury.

RELATIVE STRENGTH

Guidelines for determining the correct strength that should be demonstrated by any part of your body include three basic considerations.

Strength of the Part Relative to Your Total Body Weight

Many weight-lifting books will give standard ratios for making such a determination, or you can ask your physical therapist. Usually, these are expressed as minimum strength levels for a healthy individual. For instance, a man should be able to perform a bilateral biceps curl with weight equal to half that of his total body weight. If he cannot, either his strength needs to improve or his weight needs to be reduced. Such ratios exist for each of about a dozen different major body parts. When creating a rehabilitation program for any injured part, one way to gauge progress is when strength has returned to a level that meets these minimum requirements for health.

Strength of the Part Relative to Its Bilateral Counterpart

If you hurt your left arm, it is reasonable to assume that it has regained full strength when it is as strong as your right arm in similar movements. Most people are surprised to find that if they are left-handed they are often stronger with their right arm, and vice versa. This is because the preferred arm is the one that is used for fine motor skills such as writing, turning doorknobs or handling keys whereas the other arm is used for gross motor skills such as picking up suitcases or holding packages.

Strength of the Part Relative to Its Partner Muscle

Almost all of the muscles of the body come in opposing pairs. Most people know that they have a biceps and a triceps muscle. The biceps flexes the forearm and the triceps extends it. This is an opposing pair of muscles. Sports physiologists have developed strength ratios of one opposing muscle to the other that they find allow for optimum function of the body. Using this method, once it is determined which muscle of any opposing pair is stronger, and by how much, the results can be compared to established norms. There are suggested ratios for all of the muscle pairs of the body listed in many sports physiology books.

STATIC BEFORE DYNAMIC

Static means "not moving" when it comes to human performance. Dynamic means, "with motion." When rehabilitating any injury, ALWAYS perform static challenges to the area before attempting any dynamic challenges. The forces and variables involved in any dynamic challenge have the potential to be much greater than those associated with any static position. A static position challenges the strength of the weakest link around the involved joint: muscle, ligament, tendon, joint capsule, or even bone. Keep in mind that even though static-hold positions are safer, pressure should still be applied extremely gradually and carefully to any areas recovering from injury.

The "static before dynamic" principle is exemplified in the following example. Let's say we are trying to rehabilitate an elbow injury. Your arm has not been used for several months due to medial epicondylitis (tennis elbow). If you walk up to a bar that is at head height and grab it firmly with both hands, your elbows would be bent at about 90 degrees, their strongest position. You could then very gradually lift your weight off your feet until your weight is transferred fully to your arms. This is considered a static hold, a far less risky or challenging move to attempt than pull-ups. There are many applications to the "static before dynamic" concept. They make sense in every case.

RANGE OF MOTION

Range of motion should be explored gradually as part of the rehabilitation of any joint. The smallest possible range of motion should be attempted first, gradually building into larger movements. In the same way, the range of motion should be performed in a manner that creates the least possible stress on the joint at first, gradually increasing the stress over time as the body adapts.

In cases of rehabilitation from severe injury, the therapist may ask the patient to move the affected part with the assistance of gravity first. For instance, with a shoulder injury, the smallest range and the least resistance would be to bend forward from the waist, let the arm hang straight down, and attempt to make small, slow circles with the hand while keeping the arm straight.

Eventually, the circles could grow in size and speed. When the patient feels stronger, he or she could attempt to make circles with the arm while standing upright with the arm outstretched, parallel to the

"Range-of-motion exercises should be done extremely gently during the warm-up phase of an exercise session. Wait until the stretching and cool-down phase at the end of the session to explore the fullest ranges of motion."

"Be patient, and use slow-motion movements to test your recovery. If it hurts in slow motion, don't even think about trying to move any faster."

floor. Eventually, weight could be held in the hand, adding resistance to that already being applied by gravity.

Range-of-motion exercises should be done extremely gently during the warm-up phase of an exercise session. Wait until the stretching and cool-down phase at the end of the session to explore the fullest ranges of motion.

SLOW MOTION BEFORE FULL SPEED

When rehabilitating yourself to regain former skills, you must be careful with the injured part. Until it is fully healed, it is weaker than the surrounding parts and more prone to reinjury, and must be treated with caution accordingly.

In the following scenario, perhaps you cut yourself on the abdomen and had to take two weeks off from playing golf. Now you think you are ready to go. There is a safe way to find out.

First, very slowly and gently perform a miniature swing motion with just your arms and no club. If there is no pain or pulling from the area around the cut, you could try taking a slightly bigger swing, increasing the size of this slow movement until you are sure that there is no damage being done. Then you could try speeding up the motion. Eventually, you take a club in hand and repeat the process from the beginning, starting with small slow strokes and building their size, then their speed. If every indication shows that the wound is ready, you could then add the extra stress of actually hitting the golf ball.

A slow-motion walk-through can be done to test practically any injury. There are many injuries that will not hurt at all when walking but will cause great pain if you run. An ankle sprain will hurt even if you walk in extra slow motion at first. As it heals, you will be able to walk slowly with no pain. Eventually, you will be able to walk normally but the force of running will cause pain. Gradually you will be able to speed up your motions until you are going full speed again. Be patient, and use slow-motion movements to test your recovery. If it hurts in slow motion, don't even think about trying to move any faster.

LIMIT THE NUMBER OF VARIABLES

When focusing on rehabilitation, the fewer number of variables the better. If you are having trouble mastering a skill, you want to be able to focus on one thing at a time. Let's say you hurt your knee and are recovering nicely. You want to start a walking program to build up the strength and endurance of your knee and all the structures related to it. If perfectly smooth flat ground is not available to you, you may want to consider walking on a treadmill or in a large shopping mall. The walking surfaces they provide are smooth and regular and won't make you lose your balance, pull you aside, or put unexpected stress upon your knee. After a knee injury, it is truly amazing how sensitive it can be. A pebble, a small crack in the road, or any little bump, can put what seems like a huge force on the knee.

At this stage of rehabilitation, exercise machines are perfect. They allow you to focus on exactly the specific ability that you are trying to train while remaining completely stable in every other way. This is a huge plus when it comes to rehabilitation, for when any structure is weak due to an injury, it takes very little to cause a reinjury. By limiting the variables, you make the entire rehabilitation process much safer.

NONCONTACT RUN-THROUGHS

Long before you will be actually ready to play you will likely feel the urge to play. If your sport or fitness activity involves other people, the possibility of reinjury from a collision, accidental or otherwise, greatly increases. Create a situation where you have complete control of the playing field by beginning your training alone. Practice your moves around imaginary people. As you gain confidence, you can set cones or other objects on the field to use as obstacles in order to practice cuts and other direction changes.

When you think it is time to work out with other players, make it very clear to them that you feel vulnerable. Insist that however the game evolves, it must be a noncontact version. Even better, get everyone to consider the game as a practice. Participate in as many noncontact games as you need in order to feel comfortable before taking on the challenge of full contact.

RETURN TO TRAINING

Once you are training with your teammates, you are likely still not fully recovered. The fitness and agility that you lost is made more severe by the rustiness of your skills. If you must also be cautious because you are truly not ready to take a hit, you simply will not be able to keep up with healthy players in a game situation. Practice with your friends or teammates, but do not be in a rush to get into a game situation.

The reality is that even when you are practicing with your team, you still have to practice on your own as well. Do not cut your rehabilitation short or it might haunt you for a lifetime. Show up early for practice, as you will likely need 15 or 20 extra minutes of warm-up. Plan on taking extra time at the end to do a little more strength training and stretching than everyone else. Once you see how well everyone else moves, it will help you get a realistic assessment on how well-recovered you truly are.

RETURN TO COMPETITION

The final stage of rehabilitation from injury is your return to competition. Some people find that they return to competition as if they had never left, or do even better than they had done prior to their injury. Others find that they haven't yet reached the level of play that they hoped they had, and that competition is still more than they can handle.

If you are ready to play, congratulations are in order. Your rehabilitation was a success. Pat yourself on the back for a job well done, and remember to thank all of the people who helped you along the way. If you find that you are not yet ready, pat yourself on the back for having done so without getting hurt, and again for having come as far as you have in your rehabilitation. Even if it takes a few more weeks, months, or even another year to be back at full strength, it beats getting reinjured. Continue your training and stay focused on your goal.

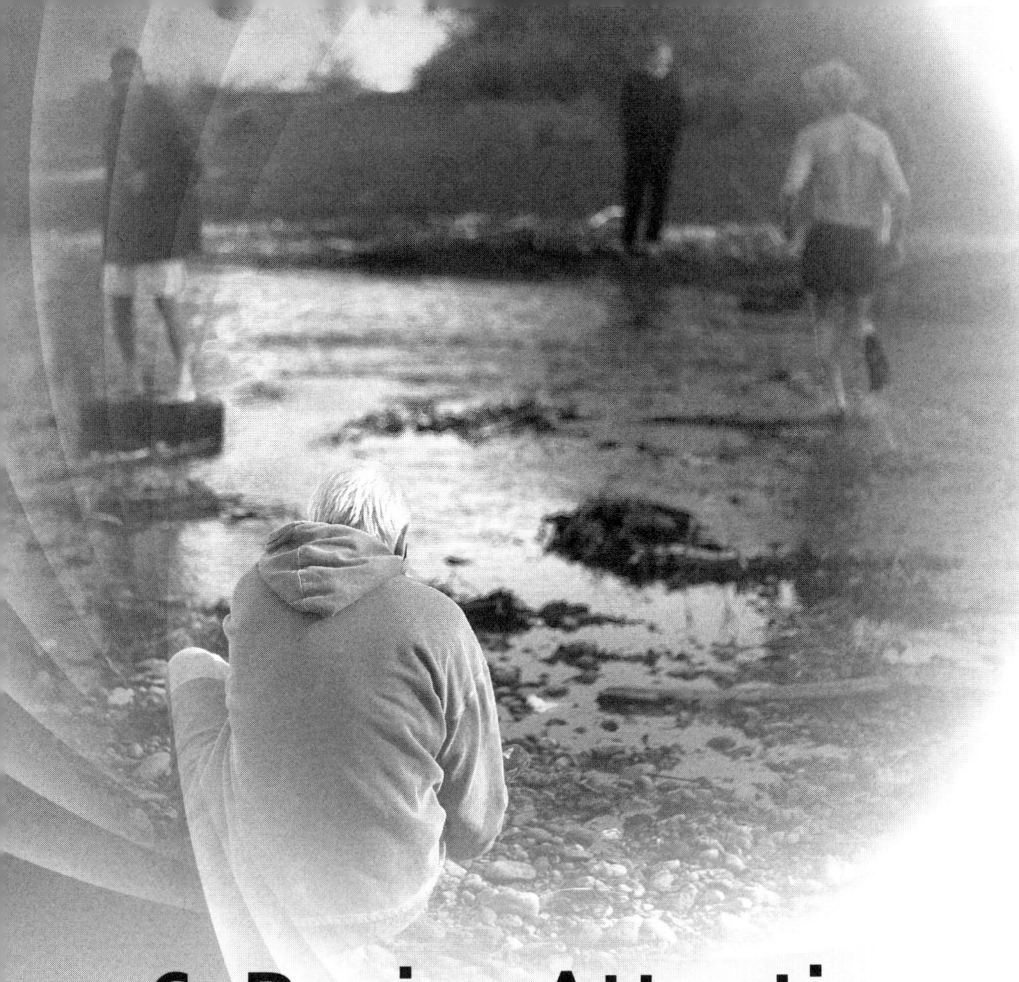

16. Paying Attention Now For a Better Future

All we have is now. An endless series of present moments pass us by, each bringing unique opportunities. When we learn from our past we can make more informed decisions, creating a better future. The best way to build a future that will be more to your liking is by increasing your awareness of the present. Gaining improved insight into the present is achieved through developing the skills that allow you to pay attention, better focus on, and truly be in the "now" moment.

MENTAL AWARENESS IS AN ASSET

Sometimes we take our mental awareness for granted. Certainly many partygoers successfully impair their mental awareness through the consumption of alcoholic beverages and recreational drugs. In sports, however, as in life, awareness is a vital asset. Awareness comes to us through our five senses and through our interpretation of the data that comes to us through those senses.

As we heighten our ability to see, touch, taste, smell, and hear, and to interpret that input, we increase our awareness of the world around us. Increased awareness equates with better decision making.

FORESIGHT IN SELF-CARE IS SMART

For some reason, we humans like to think that we are amazingly intelligent, yet we demonstrate that we are slow learners again and again. Hindsight may be 20/20, as the saying goes, but in order to truly learn from our past we must use our memory to behave more intelligently in the future. (Have you ever burned the roof of your mouth on hot pizza? More than once?) We need to demonstrate foresight if we want to experience optimum health. We must learn to recognize and avoid potentially dangerous situations before we find ourselves enmeshed in them.

REDUCE BLIND SPOTS

Very often we cannot see what we are looking for, even when it is right in front of us. This happens conceptually as well as physically. Many animals conceal themselves, using coloration and shape as effective camouflage when they are in plain sight. Much of what we need to learn about training is plain for us to see, but we generally see it much more rapidly when someone else points it out for us. One of the huge benefits of having a teacher, coach, or guide when learning any fitness activity is that they can point out the "obvious" for us. Learn from someone else's mistakes so you don't have to learn from your own.

Sometimes judgment errors are not visible until it's too late and an accident has already happened. Such is the case with the concept known as "object fixation," where you will tend to move towards that which you focus upon. While driving your car, if you have ever tried to avoid hitting something on the road by looking at it, and then hit it, you are familiar with the experience.

This occurs frequently when bicyclists attempt to ride in between tightly arranged obstacles. If they look at the obstacle they tend to hit the obstacle. Many snow skiers like to ski "off-piste" through the woods. This is often referred to as "skiing the trees," although "skiing the spaces," would, hopefully, be a more accurate description.

When it comes to our training methods, we tend to become attached to our own way of doing things and closed to new ideas, especially if they seem radical. When it comes to food, many factors cause us to resist change, including cultural training, emotional issues, habits, and social mores about right and wrong. Yet it is the overcoming of food and training blind spots that typically opens the door for many of our biggest advances in fitness performance.

OVERLOAD AND RECOVER

The application of the "overload and recover" principle is the basis of all training, and not as simple as it seems. As you become more aware, you will find new and varied ways to apply this principle successfully. The use of unstable surfaces for training, for instance, has taken the world of sport by storm. It is an excellent method of applying overload and recovery to the neurological skills aspect of training.

Sprinters run down gentle slopes (overload) to get a feel for running faster than they ever could on flat ground. Once they train their neurology to move that quickly on the slope (recovery), they can transfer the skill to flatter and eventually flat ground. The overload and recovery principle must be applied to all aspects of training if optimum performance is the desired goal.

MOMENT OF POWER

The past is over, and cannot be brought back to life. Like spilled milk, there is no point in crying about an injury that has already happened. The future is yet to come; worrying about what might happen in the future is a futile effort. Most of what we worry about (more than

90 percent according to many experts) does not come to pass. The present is the only point in time over which you can exert control. All of your power is focused in the present moment, in the now.

As you learn to pay more attention to the present, to this current moment, your power over your life, and your future, will grow. Being in the moment, "being present" as the expression goes, will hugely reduce your chances of injury as well. The more you are in the moment, the more your awareness of present conditions rises. Increased awareness means increased perception. The more present you become, the greater your vision will be.

LETTING THE PAST NEGATIVELY AFFECT THE PRESENT

It is important to learn from the past and hopefully not repeat our mistakes. Things that we perceive to have happened "ages ago" we tend to diminish in importance, especially as opposed to things that "just happened." In the midst of a tennis match, for instance, it is unlikely that you will be thinking about an unforced error that you made several years ago.

Yet if you spend more than a second or two thinking about one you "just" made, you are still giving it too much importance. Thinking about an error from two or three points ago is no more relevant than thinking about one that you made two or three years ago. This is a classic example of letting your past affect your present. It is likely that you will lose every point while you are thinking about the past instead of being in the present. In sport, it is imperative that you categorize things that have already occurred as "the past"—and keep them there. Putting the past behind you is a critical skill in all fitness activities, one that requires constant practice and reinforcement.

PRACTICE DOES NOT MAKE PERFECT

We fall into a practice routine so easily, so comfortably, and almost without thought. We allow ourselves to believe that if we just keep practicing, we will eventually get it right. It turns out that this is not the case, and what actually happens is that the skills we get better at are the skills we practice, exactly as we practice them.

This is an important part of why progressions need to be utilized in sport. If we start training with a difficult skill that we perform poorly over and over, we are also training the involved nerve pathways to allow us to do it poorly again and again. If we start training with a simple skill, one that we can master relatively easily, we can practice it perfectly time and again, training the appropriate nerve pathways as we do so.

PERFECT PRACTICE

Perfect practice makes for perfect performances. Perfect practice trains us to perform perfectly even when conditions make it more challenging. One of the biggest differences between an amateur and a professional in any sport is that an amateur practices till he or she gets it right whereas a professional practices till he or she doesn't get it wrong. Meticulousness in your training habits is healthy. The mechanics of perfect movement leave room for error without opening the door to injury. If your mechanics are poor to begin with, they invite injury.

Sloppy practices will yield sloppy performances. Make perfection your goal. Mastery is when a skill can be performed perfectly at least ten times in a row. Then it is time to embellish the skill with more detail, to move on to a more difficult version of that skill, or to begin practicing the skills for which the newly mastered skill was a lead-up.

SPECIFICITY OF TRAINING

Swimming and bicycling both can be endurance activities and both can be used to build cardiopulmonary capacity. It is highly unlikely that an athlete would train in swimming if she hoped to become a better cyclist, nor is it likely that she would be successful using that strategy. The way to become a better cyclist is by cycling. By also training in all of the related skills that play a part in cycling, such as balance, biceps strength, leg strength and power, technique, nutrition, and so on, you can insure that there are no weak links. Swimming simply would not enter into the training picture for a cyclist because the skills and abilities are almost totally unrelated.

The training effect is ultra-specific. For instance, if you train for biceps strength using an isometric contraction at 45 degrees of flexion, strength at that specific angle will increase. Such training, however, will have very little if any impact on the strength of the biceps at 90 degrees of flexion. Marathon-length runs will not result in better performances for the sprinter.

When designing your training program, it is important to know what your training goals are as well as how to train for them. The body adapts specifically to the demands that are placed on it. In other words, what you get is exactly what you train the body to do.

BEING IN THE NOW AND ZEN

There are hundreds of books on the topic of the mind-body connection in sports. The authors of *Inner Tennis, The Zen of Running, Zen in the Art of Archery, The Warrior Athlete,* and many others stress the importance of paying attention during sports, of being "in the moment." The authors stress that the only way for the body to perform at its best is when it is one with the mind, for then the mind "gets out of the way" of peak performance. There is no question that such a mindset is extremely valuable, both for the sake of performance and in injury prevention. There are many ways to achieve the goal of clear-minded attentiveness. The following methods have been proven to be extremely effective.

Visualization

Visualization is the art of rehearsing a performance in your head before actually physically attempting it. It is common to see gymnasts, springboard divers, and ice skaters visualizing their routines a few minutes before going out to perform. Often they have their eyes closed, and will use their entire body in the visualization, using their arms and legs to mock the movements they will soon be executing. When visualization is practiced at its highest levels, the nerves involved in each movement are actually engaged. In this way, visualization is practically the real thing, and in some ways it is better than the real thing. There are many advantages to using visualization.

Visualization takes up very little energy compared to the real performance and allows for much greater repetition of skills. For example, the long program in ice skating takes four minutes to perform. A skater can only practice such a routine a few times per hour, as more would be too tiring and become dangerous. However, the same skater can easily visualize the routine ten or twelve times in an hour, giving him or her plenty of chances to become aware of all the minutiae of the routine and even noting where more details are needed.

"Practicing visualization skills improves your ability to concentrate."

Visualization is completely safe and requires no special equipment. It can be practiced anywhere, at any time of day. Visualization allows for easier practicing of skill variations, different outfits, different partners, or whatever is needed, and takes far less time. Practicing your visualization skills improves your ability to concentrate while making you more familiar with your routine. Best of all, visualization is completely free.

Experience

Experience provides the opportunity to be more prepared for the future and less surprised by the unexpected. After participating in ten running races, for example, you will be far less likely to forget some little detail, such as taking your racing gear to the race. After 100 races, you will have your pre- and post-race routines down to a science. And you won't get caught with untied laces during the race, or wearing an outfit whose stitches irritate your skin. The more you feel prepared to run without having to give it any attention, the more you can pay attention to other details.

There is a lot of finesse involved in racing in general and running a race in particular. Beginners are not usually aware of what goes into creating this kind of elegance in racing, but they likely notice that the runners who finished ahead of them did *something* differently.

Starting, running in a group, running uphill and down, passing, and even finishing, all have their own specific skills. Each time you learn one of these skills, you gain experience. With every rise in experience comes increased awareness as well as ability. The more you learn, the more you see that there is to learn.

Affirmations

In the words of my dear friend and client, Mark Victor Hansen, coauthor of the *Chicken Soup for the Soul* series, "What you think about comes about." In other words, you can make your own reality come to life with your thoughts. Of course, you must put action behind your words, but, along with goals, affirmations have been the beginning of many a successful project.

Affirmations, which are essentially statements of truth, are most valuable when they are stated in a positive, objective fashion, in present time. For instance, "I have the intention, skills, ability, and equipment to run 350 miles in 2015," is a positive statement. It is objectively stated in the present tense.

Affirmations stated in a fashion that begin with the declaration of the existence of something, such as "I am," "I have," or "I make," reinforce imagery in the brain that strengthens the stated truth. Objectiveness is not a requirement for an affirmation, but it does make it easier to quantify the results. "I will learn Spanish" is a goal, whereas, "I am learning Spanish" is an affirmation. When you write your affirmations and put them in places where you are likely to see them, they bolster your perceptions of reality and help you build the future you are striving for. Affirmations work best when they are short statements.

Biofeedback

Some people really don't know how to relax their muscles. Some people aren't comfortable relaxing mentally, feeling as if they are letting down their guard, and some don't know how. Biofeedback can help. Classic biofeedback is the technique of using monitoring devices to furnish information regarding an autonomic (involuntary) bodily function, such as heart rate or blood pressure, in an attempt to gain some voluntary control over that function. Usually, graduated colored lights or sound are used to give information to the person using the biofeedback machine. With practice and some guidance, biofeedback can be a very useful learning tool.

Specific types of biofeedback also can be used to refer to information about the body that comes from the body's senses. For instance, if you are standing on a wobble board and begin to lean forward, your senses of kinesthesia, proprioception, and balance, along with your coordination, would all come into play to help you right yourself. It would be correct to say that you were getting "postural" biofeedback. Using tools to get feedback is not a new idea.

The old carnival game of hitting the springboard with a huge mallet in order to catapult a weight that would ring a bell suspended high in the air relied on technique more than brute strength. Noting how high the weight was projected on each swing of the mallet gave a rough approximation of the technique used by each person. Any type of target practice is essentially a biofeedback program. Current technology offers a wide array of biofeedback opportunities and each one of them has useful applications in the world of sports.

WHEN IS INJURY MOST LIKELY?

I was hiking in the jungle of Costa Rica with a friend. Earlier in the day we had discussed that distance was not measured in miles or kilometers in Costa Rica but in time. We had figured that in the case of an emergency, we were about two days away from the nearest help. The walking was challenging, as the paths were steep and often narrow. It seemed I was spending a lot of time looking at my feet and not taking in the wonderful scenery.

At one point, my friend, who was just a few steps ahead of me, said, "Pay attention here." I looked up and noticed that he was now standing on a narrow ledge, inching himself along. Below was a 20-foot drop into a shallow, rocky stream. His hands were inches in front of him, touching the tall sheer wall that he was passing. I appreciated his suggestion that I pay attention and was dutifully careful. Knowing when to pay attention definitely gives you a leg up when it comes to injury prevention.

First and Last Ten Minutes

I worked at a gymnastics gym for five years. Six hundred children took about 1,000 one-hour classes each week, and about 50 team members took five two-hour classes per week. We kept track of all injuries. During that entire time, in over 250,000 classes, fully 90 percent of all injuries happened during the first and last ten minutes of class. The reasons for this were discussed in the sections on warm-up and cool-down in Chapter 1.

The main reason that people get hurt at the beginning and end of a workout session is because they are not paying attention. Knowing that these are the absolute prime times to experience an injury should help encourage you to be a little more cautious during your warm-up and by planning for an appropriate cool-down.

When You Are Tired

Any time you are tired it becomes more difficult to pay attention. If you have not been getting enough sleep, it is important to make allowances for your tiredness when planning the duration, intensity, and frequency of your training each day. In addition, physical tiredness can come upon you rapidly during fitness activities. Be sure to plan for recovery from intense training, both during and after your workout. If you are so tired that you cannot muster your usual level of intensity or your exercising does not feel valuable, you are likely far better off to begin your cool-down and call it a day. There is always tomorrow, if you don't get hurt today.

> **"There is always tomorrow, if you don't get hurt today."**

If It Is Not Interesting, You Will Not Pay Attention

When your attention lags, you are prone to making silly mistakes. Many talented people experience this when they play a game or sport with beginners. They tend to make the same mistakes the beginners are making. Because playing with a beginner is not challenging, the more advanced player can easily become distracted from the game. Regardless of the level of play, it is important to remain focused on the game. Find a way to make every fitness session interesting. When bodies are in motion, pay attention.

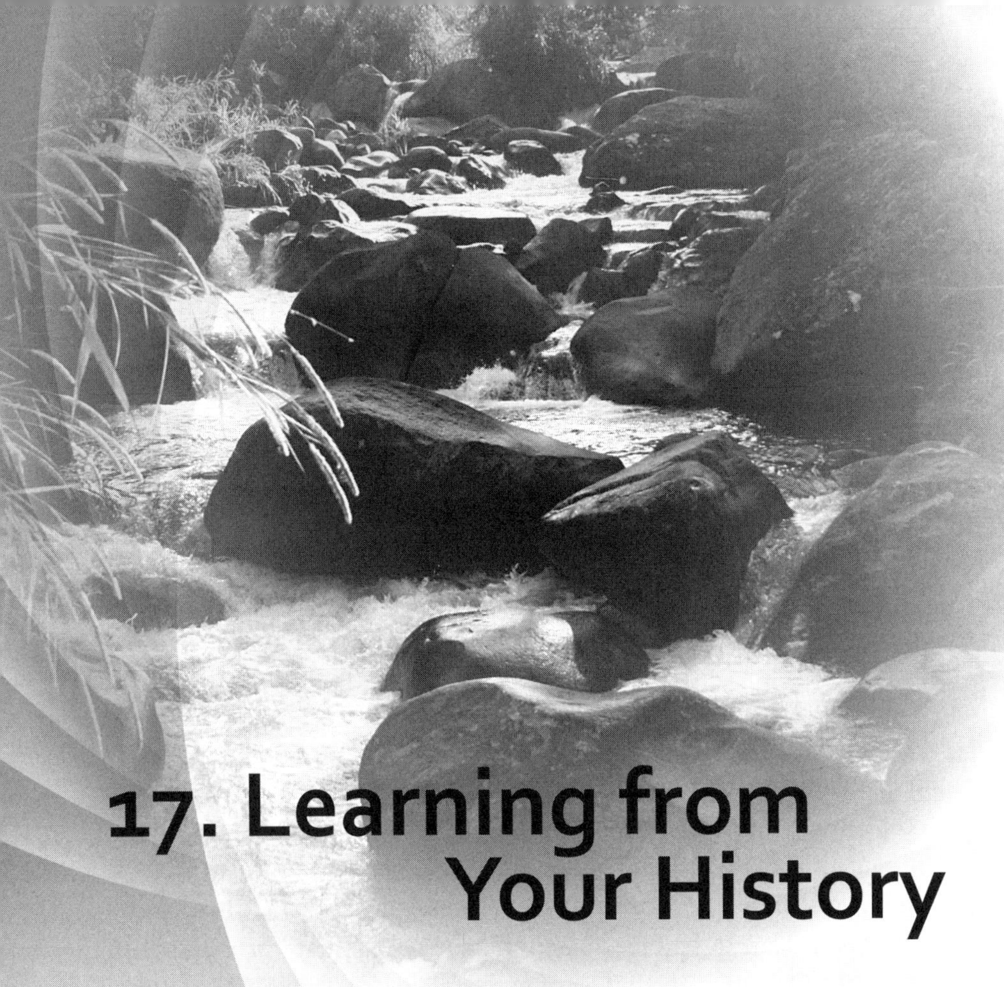

17. Learning from Your History

Each experience pertaining to training or recovering adds another piece to the puzzle of a successful fitness practice. Over time, you can accumulate a complete picture of what your ideal training program should embody. Of course, there are certain general considerations and modifications that must be made for each passing decade of life and as injuries accrue. For the most part, however, learning from your personal fitness experiences will greatly augment what you can learn from others.

There are many significant lessons to be learned in sports, and coaches help to make those lessons more obvious and more meaningful. You are much more likely to notice the important "bits and pieces" about training if you have been guided in advance to look for them. Determining the meaning of each lesson must remain up to individual interpretation. The following information provides guidelines and insights for getting the most out of your lifetime of fitness experience.

"Although it is useful to be blessed with good foresight, it is imperative to develop excellent hindsight. Without it, we are destined to repeat our mistakes again and again."

DÉJÀ VU

Everyone experiences injury from time to time and no one enjoys having the same injury time and again. That is one déjà vu experience that we can all live without. Likewise, when we have peak experiences in athletics, we don't simply want to repeat them, we hope to improve upon them. Although it is useful to be blessed with good foresight, it is imperative to develop excellent hindsight. Without it, we are destined to repeat our mistakes again and again.

Learning from our mistakes does not mean that we will cease making mistakes. There are countless mistakes to be made, and many of them turn out to be blessings in disguise. The main problem with repeating a mistake is that it doesn't take long to train the nerve pathways involved, thus creating a habit of making the mistake.

When you hear someone say, "Darn, I always do that," they are usually referring to making a mistake that has become habitual. There are methods for preventing errors from becoming habits and ways to break such habits if they already exist.

THE VALUE OF HINDSIGHT

When you are in the midst of a fitness activity, especially a competitive one, time to think is usually at a premium. There is barely enough time to act let alone make a mental note. And in the course of a game such as tennis, keeping track of such things can be distracting, keeping you from focusing on the match at hand. Fortunately, we spend considerably more time in practice than we do in competition. The "rules" during practice are much more lenient.

Depending upon the activity, it will probably be considered acceptable behavior if you need to write a quick note to yourself now and then during a training session in order to remember something that will help your performance. It is likely that your partners, coaches, teammates, and even your competitors want you to improve in your skills, and they will usually make little allowances for your quirks during a practice session.

Obviously some activities lend themselves to this more than others. Creating a mental or written list of errors that you wish to improve upon or correct will prove extremely valuable and provide fodder for some of the most useful training sessions you will ever undertake.

STUDY YOUR MISTAKES

We all make mistakes in technique, mechanics, judgment, and strategy. Accepting your mistakes is a part of good sportsmanship. Studying your mistakes demonstrates your interest and motivation in improving yourself and your game. Correcting your mistakes is an important part of how you become a better player.

It wasn't very long ago that the only way you could study your mistakes was by thinking about them or by asking someone else to watch and evaluate your performance. Today's technology allows you to view your performance instantly and make the necessary corrections accordingly.

"Creating a mental or written list of errors that you wish to improve upon or correct will prove extremely valuable and provide fodder for some of the most useful training sessions you will ever undertake."

STUDY THE PROS

As the level at which the top performers in any sport improves, the level of play goes up throughout the ranks of players. Since we often copy the "moves" of the stars, when fewer mistakes are made by the top people, there are fewer mistakes for us to copy. As soon as new moves or improvements in mechanics are developed by our sports heroes, the kids on the street start practicing them. There is no wonder about why the level of sports performance continues to rise.

There are several tried and true methods for overcoming specific errors in sports performance, especially those that have already become habit.

Slow Motion

Reflex decisions and actions can be flawed. Sometimes, correct mechanics or tactical responses need to be learned. By slowing down the action, we can practice making the correct responses exactly as we want them to be. This technique works just as well for footwork as it does for strategy. Learn to perform in slow motion, and as it becomes less awkward, gradually speed up the movements. Eventually, the correct response will feel automatic and you will be able to perform it at full speed.

De-Stress by Isolating the Situation

During the middle of a game or match is not the time to try to learn new behavior. To really make the most of a learning situation, remove as many variables as possible and simply focus on the one behavior you are trying to embrace. Break complex movements into their component parts, and then learn each part.

"To really make the most of a learning situation, remove as many variables as possible and simply focus on the one behavior you are trying to embrace."

Over time, you will be able to link the parts, first in slow motion and eventually at game pace. If you find yourself stumbling at any point in a learning process, you are likely taking on too much at once or trying to do it too fast. Slow down and separate each aspect of a skill from the others. Once you learn them properly you will find that joining them in sequence is much easier.

Repeat the "Feel" of Doing It Right

Every once in a while things just "click" in an athletic endeavor and you outperform your expectations. Usually when this happens, you actually were not trying as hard as customary. Try to remember what it felt like, or to find any other clues as to what you just did, and then attempt to repeat that performance.

Sometimes you "just know" that you were on to something, and it is worth taking the time, right then, to try to master that aspect of your performance. Once you get the feel of doing something correctly, it gets increasingly easy to do it that way almost every time.

While it can be initially confusing to try to "not try," that is exactly what you must do if you want to effortlessly perform well. Once you learn proper mechanics, the act of thinking about what you are doing while you are doing it will only hinder your performance. A common problem in sports, this phenomenon is called "getting in your own way." Your goal should be to perform without thinking about it, automatically. If you have to analyze your movements while performing them, you need more practice.

The Value of Skills and Drills

Every fitness activity is partly composed of a variety of specific skills. These skills are usually either extremely simple or able to be broken down into a series of basic components. Learning these skills or their component parts is achieved through the practice of drills. Drills are used to reduce the number of variables and focus the desired outcome for any specific skill. For instance, there are many ways to hit a forehand shot in tennis. There is the topspin, backspin, cross-court, inside-out, down-the-line, and many other forehand shots. Each one is a separate skill and there are a variety of drills for learning each of them.

Drills can be very rewarding to practice on their own. Some people find playing their sport to be the most fun and consider performing repetitive drills to be boring. Others find that doing the drills is as rewarding and sometimes more fun than playing the sport itself. For instance, the game of tennis can be very slow. The points can be short, and for beginners, a great many mistakes are made. More time is spent between points than on them. Practicing a drill can provide the opportunity for much more tennis play than the actual game does. Most of us need more practice and repetition than we give ourselves time to do. We would benefit tremendously by putting more time into practicing the drills and mastering the skills, even if it means less time actually playing the sport.

For people who find drills boring, I recommend making a game or competition out of them. If you are practicing serves in tennis, two or more people can practice serving at the same time. The first person to get ten serves in is the winner. Almost every drill provides the option of keeping score, racing, or somehow making it competitive. They also offer a chance to practice cooperatively.

Cooperative drills, such as seeing how long you can keep a rally going, provide an excellent opportunity to repeat a skill (or skills) and embrace the very nature of teamwork that is so important to many sports and activities. The more that a workout can be turned into a play session, the more enthusiasm you are likely to put into it and the more enjoyment you are likely to get out of it. If you know that you like to play but that workouts can be boring for you, turn your work into play and have fun doing drills.

"The more that a workout can be turned into play, the more enthusiasm you are likely to put into it and the more enjoyment you are likely to get out of it."

Broaden Neuro Capabilities

Each time you learn a new skill or way of moving, it requires the training of nerve pathways. While it is possible that your use of that movement will be forever and always restricted to a particular sports activity, it is far more likely that you will see applications for it in other endeavors as well. This crossover of movements from one sport to another also brings benefits into our everyday life in two ways.

To illustrate the first benefit, let's say that you learned a split step as part of a soccer drill (though it is also used in tennis and other sports). A few days later, to keep from bumping into someone in a busy store, you might just use that split step. As for the second benefit, each time you train a new nerve pathway you enhance the function of the others. Regaining your balance as you almost fall down a flight of stairs you might (rightly) think to yourself that all of the coordination training you have been doing of late, including learning the split step, saved you from taking a bad fall.

Recognize Patterns

There are many similar movements that transfer from sport to sport. Running uphill is much like cycling or speed skating, in-line skating is closely related to snow skiing, and surfing, skateboarding, and water skiing on one ski all use skills that are very similar to each other. As you learn more skills, the related movement patterns will become apparent to you.

Recognizing that a new skill is not that different from one with which you are already familiar makes it much easier to learn. Insights about the skill, variations on the skill, and ways to practice it, all come more easily if you can see or feel a movement pattern within it that already is familiar to you.

COORDINATION LEADS TO STREAMLINED PERFORMANCE

Filling in the gaps of missing skills using the drills that make learning them easiest also results in a more streamlined performance. As you refine your movements due to practicing drills, extraneous motion is eliminated and you become more coordinated. Your newly coordinated movements focus your efforts more powerfully, and require less exertion than the earlier versions. It is interesting and rewarding to note that not only is performance enhanced as movements become more coordinated but safety increases dramatically as well.

CHRONIC INJURIES NEED TO BE ADDRESSED

Though historians teach that "history repeats itself" there is no reason that injuries need to be chronic. In fact, if you are constantly repeating the same injury again and again, something needs to change. Your body can handle abuse (though abuse takes its toll in terms of health losses) but it is designed to function optimally when it is extremely well cared for. Injuries are to be avoided, and the cause of chronic injuries needs to be addressed.

YOUR PARTS ARE FINITE

Our bodies are different from machines. Machines wear out from use. We grow and develop with use, and wear out from disuse, misuse, and abuse. Our parts are finite, but their functional life is greatly shortened when injuries come into the picture. Parts that should last two or three hundred years might last only twenty or thirty when they are continually damaged. Like a tire that is out of alignment, our parts can wear away to nothing, in an extremely short time, when abused. Perhaps the most rapid decay of the body and its abilities occurs when it is not used at all. Disuse is a death sentence to the body or to any specific part of the body.

Take care of your body and it will likely function well throughout a long and healthy lifetime. Misuse, disuse, or abuse your body and you will pay with pain, suffering, lost health and reduced ability to function, for the price of health is not negotiable.

"Take care of your body and it will likely function well throughout a long and healthy lifetime."

CORRECTING THE CAUSE

It is always healthier to remove the cause of a problem than it is to supplement the problem. If you are tired, getting more sleep is a healthier solution than using stimulants. You might use an interim program while you are correcting the cause of your health or injury concerns, but this must be considered a stop-gap measure at best. Chronic injuries must be addressed, and at their cause, or they will continue to occur. The price in wear and tear is more than anyone can take, but it does not stop there.

There is pain, suffering, downtime, rehabilitation time, and missed fun. There are all of the related activities that must be skipped, and the sheer energy of deciding what is, and what is not, a safe enough activity to attempt. With every recurrence of a chronic injury, there is some degree of self-belittling. Issues concerning self respect invariably come up with chronic injuries, as does the issue of being a "whole" person. Whether the cause of your chronic injury is nutritional, functional, physical, or tactical, address the cause fully and correct it. The sooner the better with such injuries, for each injury adds another straw to break the proverbial camel's back.

STRENGTHEN WEAK LINKS

Once the cause of chronic injury has been corrected, it is imperative that the weakest links of your fitness program be addressed. These may or may not have to do directly with the chronic injury. If they do, correcting them will bolster and support recovery making the same injury much less likely to happen in the future. If your weak links are not directly related to a chronic injury, they are likely setting the stage for another injury to happen. As you strengthen the weak links of your health and fitness program, you will experience both specific and general improvements in your health and fitness performance. The effort is therefore extremely rewarding, making it a practice that you will want to continue throughout your lifetime.

TRAIN SMARTER TO TRAIN HARDER

Smart training means getting the most out of your fitness activities. It means being able to increase the frequency, intensity, and even the duration of your training as you see fit, without having recovery problems. Smart training means staying injury-free. It means being able to train more each year, if you wish to, and being able to be active for your entire life. Training smarter results in improved performance abilities on every level.

EXTEND YOUR SEASON, EXTEND YOUR CAREER

Consider the warm-up and cool-down as essentials in your smart training regimen. Use the warm up and cool down with every workout and you will notice that your recovery improves. Smart training includes smart recovering. As you improve your abilities to monitor and support speedy recovery, your enthusiasm and ability to train will increase. You will find that you can train more days per year due to your improved recovery regimen.

Improving your nutrition is another facet of smart training. By increasing the percentage of whole, fresh, ripe, raw, organic fruits and vegetables in your diet, you will become more energetic and less injury prone. The newfound energy will result in workouts that are more valuable. By becoming less prone to injury you will find that you can increase the amount of life in your workouts and the number of workouts in your life.

KEEPING IT FRESH AND FUN

Smart training requires variety. Long before any activity can become boring, you should switch to a new one. Use every aspect of variety that you can think of, including watching how other people train and trying their way. We are prone to falling in a rut with our exercises. Train with different people now and then. Go to a new location to work out. Play a different game than the ones you are used to or good at. If you usually play singles, try some doubles. If you are a lefty, play right-handed, at least once in a while. Fitness is for fun. Instead of focusing your training on the functional fitness that it provides, try training once a month purely for the joy of the fact that you *can* train. It is perfectly acceptable to be a beginner at any sport or activity, so keep trying new ones. Go out and play, like you did when you were a kid, and take the work out of your workouts.

INJURY-FREE IS THE WAY TO GO

Injuries end the fun of training. As you train smarter, it becomes more fun-filled and less painful. When injury-free, training is a joy. You can train because you want to rather than because you have to. When you are injury-free, you can choose your activities rather than having to do something specifically for its rehabilitative value. When you train smarter, you train as if your life depended upon it. Eating, sleeping, warming up and cooling down, working out, and recovering, all support your ability to remain injury-free. When you are injury-free, the joy of movement will want make you want to train for the rest of your life, and you will become able to do so.

AVOID CAREER-ENDING MISTAKES

Some accidents that happen are simply out of our control. Most of the time, however, we cause them all by ourselves. Training smart means being able to see and avoid these potential pitfalls. Career-ending injuries are often devastating surprises. Trust your judgment and trust your senses. You don't have to get hurt in order to know that certain activities are dangerous. Nor do you have to avoid any physical pursuit. If you intend to participate in a dangerous sport or game, take lessons from a pro and wear the appropriate protective gear. Plan to play for the rest of your life.

"Training smart means being able to see and avoid potential pitfalls."

CATER TO YOUR UNIQUENESS

Every well-known athlete is famous because of his or her unique qualities. Some golfers are known for their putting, others for their driving. Some are considered great because of their accuracy, or the well-rounded nature of their game. Each of them has something that makes them unique, as do we all. Develop your weak areas and you will become better at your chosen fitness activities. Develop your strengths and you will stand out for them.

USE WHAT YOU KNOW ABOUT YOURSELF

No one knows you better than yourself. Use that knowledge to motivate yourself to be your best and you will increase your joy and participation in fitness activities. If you know you respond well to coaching, use a coach with regularity. If you are a visual learner, watch the great ones perform and follow their visual model. If you know that you tend to cut your warm-ups short, make every effort to extend them. You know your strengths and you know your weaknesses. Provide yourself with the conditions, influences, substances, and forces that give you the best opportunity to reach your fullest fitness potential.

GROW IN EVERY WAY THAT YOU CAN

Many people underestimate their abilities and never discover or develop their true potential. Our preconceived notions of sports performance can be limiting in their scope. There is room for everyone, and for everyone to learn. Every experience can be a growth experience. Open yourself to life's possibilities and follow its opportunities. Learning is more than a fundamental part of life. Learning is fun.

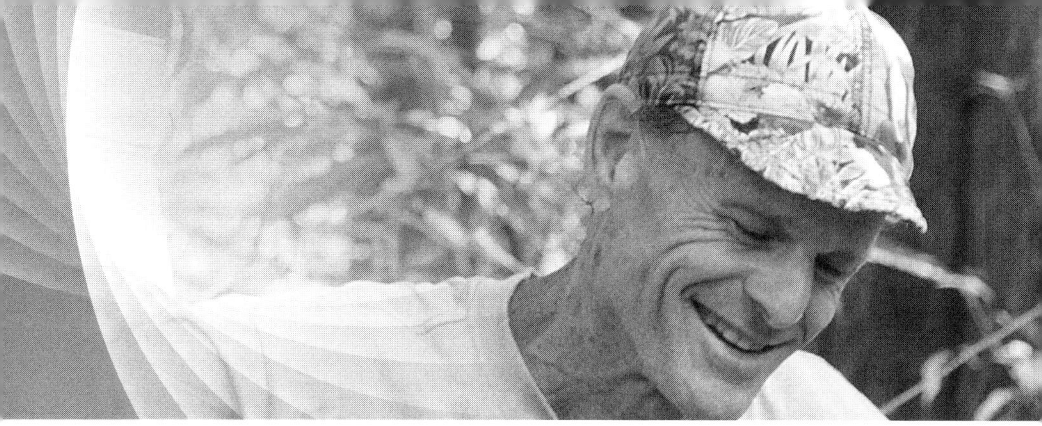

ABOUT THE AUTHOR

DR. DOUGLAS GRAHAM, a lifetime athlete and raw fooder since the Seventies, is an advisor to world-class athletes and trainers from around the globe. After competing as a collegiate gymnast and internationally on the trampoline, and coaching seven national trampoline champions, he now works professionally with top performers from almost every sport and field of entertainment. Some of these include such notables as tennis legend Martina Navratilova, NBA pro basketball player Ronnie Grandison, track Olympic sprinters Doug Dickinson and Isa Philips, pro women's soccer player Callie Withers, championship bodybuilder Kenneth G. Williams, *Chicken Soup for the Soul* coauthor Mark Victor Hansen (who credits Dr. Graham with having saved his career,) and actress Demi Moore.

Dr. Graham is the author of several books on raw food and health, including *The High Energy Diet Recipe Guide, Nutrition and Athletic Performance, The 80/10/10 Diet,* and the forthcoming *Perpetual Health.*

The 80/10/10 Diet, currently being translated into more than 20 languages, has spawned many international festivals based on its precepts, and helped grow the raw food movement by providing effective, health-promoting, and sports-enhancing dietary advice that thousands have embraced.

Dr. Graham has shared his strategies for success with audiences at more than 4,000 presentations worldwide. Recognized as one of the fathers of the raw movement, Dr. Graham is the only lecturer to have attended and given keynote presentations at all of the major raw events in the world, from 1997 through 2005, and he continues to give keynote presentations at raw festivals the world over.

He is the creator of "Simply Delicious" cuisine, and the director of Health & Fitness Weeks, which provide Olympic-class training and nutritional guidance to people of all fitness levels in beautiful settings around the world. He is living proof that eating whole, fresh, ripe, raw, organic food is the nutritional way to vibrant health and vitality.

BIBLIOGRAPHY

Airola, Paavo O. *How to Get Well: Dr. Airola's Handbook of Natural Healing.* Phoenix, AZ: Health Plus Publishers, 1984.

Bowsher, David. *Introduction to the Anatomy & Physiology of the Nervous System,* 3rd ed. Oxford: Blackwell Scientific Publishers, 1975.

Chusid, Joseph G. *Correlative Neuroanatomy & Functional Neurology,* 16th ed. Los Altos, CA: Lange Medical Publications, 1976.

Coleman, John. 1998. Opioids in Common Food Products: Addictive Peptides in Meat, Dairy and Grains. http://www. karlloren.com/diet/p18.htm.

Cornish, J.L. MD., *Health Knowledge.* New York: Medical Book Distributors. 1947

DeVries, Herbert A. *Physiology of Exercise for Physical Education and Athletics.* Dubuque, IA: William C. Brown Company, 1966.

Fry, T.C., *Better Sleep for a Better Life,* Life Science Society, 1976.

Gray, Henry. *Anatomy, Descriptive and Surgical,* 15th ed. T. Pickering Pick & Robert Howden, Eds. New York: Bounty Books, 1977.

Groff, James L. and Susan S. Gropper. *Advanced Nutrition and Human Metabolism.* 3rd ed. Belmont, CA: Wadsworth, 2000.

Heritage, Ford. *Composition and Facts about Foods and Their Relationship to the Human Body.* Pomeroy, WA: Health Research, 1971.

Jacobs, David S., Bernard L. Kasten, Jr., Wayne R. Demott, and William L. Wolfson. *Laboratory Test Handbook,* 2nd ed. Hudson, OH: Lexi-Comp, 1990.

Johnson, Perry and Donald Stolberg. *Conditioning.* Englewood Cliffs, NJ: Prentice-Hall, 1971.

McAlpine, Ken. *Eat To Compete. American Way. Sept. 1999: 56-134. Print.*

McArdle, William D., Frank I. Katch, and Victor L. Katch. *Exercise Physiology: Energy, Nutrition, and Human Performance,* 3rd ed. Philadelphia: Lea & Febiger, 1986.

Onywera, VO. et al. "Food and macronutrient intake of elite kenyan distance runners." Int J Sport Nutr Exerc Metab. 2004 Dec;14(6):709-19.

Time-Life Books. *Restoring the Body: Treating Aches and Injuries.* Alexandria, VA: Time-Life Education, 1987.

First Aid Manual: The Authorised Manual of St. John Ambulance, St. Andrew's Ambulance Association and The British Red Cross, 8th ed. London: Dorling Kindersley Publishers, 2006.

Read, Malcolm and Paul Wade. *Sports Injuries: A Unique Self-Diagnosis and Treatment Guide.* London: Breslich & Foss, 1984.

Shelton, Herbert M. *Orthopathy.* Natural Hygiene Press, 1980.

Shelton, Herbert M. *The History of Natural Hygiene and Principles of Natural Hygiene* Whitefish: Kessinger Publishing. 2010

Tortora, Gerard J. *Introduction to the Human Body: The Essentials of Anatomy and Physiology.* 2nd ed. New York: HarperCollins, 1991.

Tortora, Gerard J. and Sandra Reynolds Grabowski. *Principles of Anatomy and Physiology.* 5th ed. New York: John Wiley & Sons, 2001.

Wells, Katharine F. and Kathryn Luttgens. *Kinesiology: Scientific Basis of Human Motion,* 7th ed. Philadelphia: Saunders College Publishing, 1982.

Williams, Thomas R., *The Laws of Vital Relation.* Self Published, 1985.

Wilson, Kathleen J.W. *Ross and Wilson Anatomy and Physiology in Health and Illness,* 6th ed. New York: Churchill Livingstone, 1987.